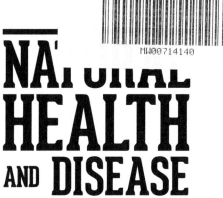

NATURAL HEALTH AND DISEASE PREVENTION

NATURAL HEALTH AND DISEASE PREVENTION

Alfred Anduze M.D

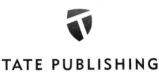

TATE PUBLISHING
AND ENTERPRISES, LLC

Published by Tate Publishing & Enterprises, LLC
127 E. Trade Center Terrace | Mustang, Oklahoma 73064 USA
1.888.361.9473 | www.tatepublishing.com

Tate Publishing is committed to excellence in the publishing industry. The company reflects the philosophy established by the founders, based on Psalm 68:11,
"The Lord gave the word and great was the company of those who published it."

Book design copyright © 2016 by Tate Publishing, LLC. All rights reserved.
Cover design by Dante Rey Redido
Interior design by Gram Telen

Published in the United States of America

ISBN: 978-1-68319-605-1
1. Health & Fitness / Diseases / General
2. Health & Fitness / Diet & Nutrition / General
16.07.05

This book is dedicated to A. Adelbert Anduze, scholar, teacher, lawyer, writer, musician, entertainer, and brother extraordinaire. I am sorry that your ordeal with MM was so merciless and painful and that we were so busy with the business of medicine that the simple notion of prevention was completely overlooked. Your life was full of purpose and meaning. And to my dear wonderful mother, Arminthia Elizabeth Anduze nee Lee, who succumbed to and remained locked in the chambers of Alzheimer's at a time when we neither knew nor did anything to prevent dementia. You did not deserve such an early call to the grave.

And this is for Aubrey Anduze, Bernard Elwin, Richard Bell, Madeleine Anduze, Gregory Anduze, and Catherine Anduze. If only we had been aware of and been able to follow the basic strategies toward good health as outlined in this book, perhaps your lives would have been extended and their quality improved.

May you all rest in peace.

Acknowledgments

The contents of this book are based upon the principles of medicine, the basic strategies of disease prevention, evidence-based medicine, and the vision of Andrew Weil, MD, the pioneer of integrative medicine.

Sincere appreciation goes to Miles Galin, MD, for his deep wisdom in all things medical and most things global. The scope of his knowledge and interpretation of the scientific world is a steadfast support for this work.

Thank you to Frank J. Cook, MD, on respiratory pathology.

Thank you to Dante Galiber, MD, on cardiovascular and issues on internal medicine.

Thank you to Jose Mendez-Coll, MD, on dermatology.

Thank you to Walter Pedersen, MD, on bone health and orthopedics.

Thank you to Ronald Anders, MD, on women's health.

Thank you to John Merritt, MD, for his expertise on eye care.

It is a pleasure to work with and to express my gratitude to Selena Anduze-Anaya for her motivation, advice, and professional editing.

Contents

Preface

This book was written for the general public as well as students and health care providers of all levels to explore the avenues of preventive medicine and see that "prevention *is* better than cure." After forty years of conventional medical practice, it is increasingly apparent to me (and many others) that the current health care system of treating sick people with strong and toxic pharmaceuticals, interventional and sometimes unnecessary surgery, and complex technological procedures is not working very well. Unfortunately, we tend to wait until an illness is well established before giving it attention.

In addition, the practice of medicine has changed dramatically and drastically and we, as physicians, no longer provide a service to individuals and care to patients. Instead, we follow protocols to arrive at diagnoses then implement treatments of dubious effect and with sometimes life-threatening consequences, with the benefits often flowing to entities other than the patient.

Many burdensome rules and regulations direct us away from patient care and toward business and profit motives as seen with in the dispensation of drugs and performance of interventional surgeries that are not always in the best interest of the patient.

We fear our colleagues, detest some of our patients, and are indifferent to the big organizations we call hospitals as they run our lives and sometimes ruin the lives of our patients, literally and financially. As luck and geography would have it, I was able to call upon a strong background in and respect for traditional medicine in much of my patient management. At a very young age, while growing up on the island of St. Croix in the Virgin Islands, I was often grasped gently by the hand and led into a field of wonderful plants and flowers and trees. Margaret Ortiz, my after-kindergarten caretaker, would identify and gather various plants for medicinal purposes and allow me to help.

There were leaves for upset tummy and ladies' health, fruit for sugar, flowers for blood pressure, roots for sleeping, and berries to help people love you, though I am still trying hard to remember the name of the last one. Ms. Margaret lived to a healthy old age and enjoyed the company of a handsome husband who was faithful and attentive to the end.

Always content, she had concocted, arranged, and managed a way of life that gave her both quality and longevity based on simple practical strategies that worked. It was my duty, honor, and pleasure to write this book to provide the medical world and the general public with natural methods and products in the prevention and management of disease, some of which I am sure Ms. Margaret had put to good use many years ago.

Preventive medicine makes much more sense than interventional medicine.

How to use this book: When the doctor and staff tell you early on, that you might be susceptible to a disease condition, or when you are told at the end, that there is nothing more that can be done for your condition, consider that there are multiple options for preventing the condition and for altering its course once established. It is always worth a try.

Read through chapters 1 and 2 for the general meaning and purpose of preventive medicine. Identify the condition(s) of interest in chapter 3 and examine the products assigned to that condition(s). Each is listed alphabetically, with its primary contents, mode of action, use, dosage, and side effects, if any. Find the same condition in chapter 4 and note the specific strategies recommended for prevention and natural treatment.

Though the contents, the information provided, and the suggestions are in no way intended to replace conventional diagnosis and treatment, they are evidence-based, well-tested methods, and strategies directed toward achieving and maintaining a healthy lifestyle and sense of well-being through integrative medicine and common sense.

—Alfred L. Anduze, MD, 2015

Introduction

You are responsible for your own health.

> Almost all disease conditions are preventable. Choosing to lead a healthy lifestyle will result in a better quality of life and increased longevity.
>
> —Alfred L. Anduze, MD

Becoming and staying healthy is the subject of this book. Much of the information you need to make healthy choices is contained within the pages that follow. The aim of a well-managed life is to remain in good health, avoid conditions that require long-term pharmaceutical drugs or expensive procedures and maintain one's senses and cognition into advanced age. Having seen my parents and many of my patients lose their basic physiological functions due to preventable disorders, I am convinced that with certain lifestyle adjustments, one can enter into and navigate "old age" with most systems intact. So far, at sixty-seven years of age, I have been blessed with fairly good health as evident by lack of dependence on any pharmaceuticals and have escaped any major surgical procedures. I believe this has been accomplished largely through implementations of basic strategies of lifestyle: exercise, nutrition, social connections, mental stimulation, stress reduction, and avoidance of risky behavior. I welcomed and participated in all sports since age ten and never stopped moving; I eat local and organic the majority of the time, and revere family, acquire new and maintain established friends, reading, writing, and voraciously pursuing information on all that interests me. It is a conscious effort to reduce stress by intensely effective management and avoidance of all forms of toxic exposure and activity. As a firm believer in "every little bit helps," attention to detail appears to give positive results. In avoiding the big four (heart disease, cancer, obesity, and diabetes), one's entry into old age offers better chances of a clean, comfortable exit when the time arrives.

All preventive practices and natural health products introduced and discussed are compliant with evidence-based medicine. The ultimate goal is to promote wellness, prevent illness, and alleviate the restrictions of chronic diseases, through integrative medicine, and the combination of all available and effective forms of prevention, diagnosis, and treatment.

Let us start with an overview of the status of disease in the modern era. The first challenge to our health status in the United States.[*]

---

[*] National Health and Nutrition Examination Survey (NHANES) Source: Ogden C.L. et al 2014 Prevalence of childhood and adult obesity in the United States (2011–2012).

The first challenge is the current status of disease in the modern era.[†]

1. 10.3% of individuals in the USA of all ages are in fair to poor health.

2. The leading causes of death in the USA are the following:

    1. Heart disease

    2. Cancer

    3. Chronic respiratory diseases

    4. Stroke (*cerebrovascular)*

    5. Accidents (*trauma, drug overdoses*)

    6. Alzheimer's/dementia

    7. Diabetes

    8. Infectious pneumonia/influenza (*poor immunity*)

    9. Nephritis/nephropathy (*renal failure*)

    10. Suicide (*associated with mental imbalance*)
        70-80% of these are preventable by making the correct lifestyle choices.

3. 40-50% of mortality/morbidity is associated with environmental toxicity.

†

4.   18% of 18 year olds smoke cigarettes.

5.   22% of eighteen-year-olds admitted to having had five or more drinks in one day over the past year.

6.   Obesity is strongly associated with chronic inflammation and affects the following:

   a.   8.4% of children between the ages of 2 to 5

   b.   17.7% of children between the ages of 6 to11

   c.   20.5% of teens between the ages of 12 to 19

   d.   35.1% of those over the age of 20

7.   Hypertension affects 32.5% of those over the age of twenty.

As an ophthalmic surgeon involved primarily with health of the eye, my concerns were centered on cataracts, glaucoma, diabetic retinopathy, infections, trauma, and macular degeneration. As time progressed, our care for these disorders did not change, nor did they significantly affect the outcomes. The percent of cataract patients with diabetes doubled over thirty years, half were overweight or obese, and one out of three had some degree of arthritic aches, pains, and dysfunction. Glaucoma leads to blindness at the same steady rate as before, and new and more effective treatments for diabetic retinopathy appeared to be neutralized by the increase in diabetic cases leading to irreversible blindness. What were physicians and pharmacologists and technologists doing to stem the increase? Could it all be attributed to a population growing older and a little bit more reckless? After seeing the Swiss doctors do FRAS levels (antioxidants) on all their patients, I started doing C-reactive protein (CRP) levels on preoperative patients and found that a huge number (75%)—three out of four—registered high. The level of inflammation in the bodies of my patients was certainly influencing their dysfunctional conditions and outcomes. As a comprehensive practitioner, I encountered traumatic as well as cosmetic cases. The ease and facility of operating on "healthy" tissue and watching it heal properly was so apparent that I rapidly preferred these cases to the complex, potentially complicated cases of my beloved "more unhealthy" patients. Inflammation associated with lifestyle choices, some dictated by economic, environment, and availability, others by lack of awareness and motivation to pursue a healthier line, and still others by tradition. The Caribbean penchant for eating as a sport, wherein a healthy plate of food contains three starches, a pile of red meat complete with gravy, a smattering of vegetables, with large piece of cake closely attached, and washed down with a huge sweet punch or juice, continues to baffle me (and others). Somehow, modern technology correlates and fosters lack of physical activity. Walking to a destination, no matter how near, is a thing of the past. People may still sit together, but prefer to stare at and punch letters on a cell phone rather than make eye contact or speak verbally to each other. Meanwhile the stressors mount up and accumulate, and the chemistry of resolution continues to be promoted.

What have we or are we doing to prevent these unhealthy practices that promote obscene levels of inflammation? Physicians need to take the lead in educating the population on basic health strategies as well as set a good example on exactly how to implement them.

The second challenge to the state of modern health care is our treatment approach, which sometimes does more harm than good.

8. An estimated 120 people die daily from legal and illegal drug overdose, another seven thousand people are treated in the ER for misuse or abuse of drugs, and one hundred thousand die each year from reactions to properly prescribed medications.

9. Drug overdose kills more people (twenty-five to sixty-four years old) than motor vehicle accidents (MVA). Of these, 81 percent are unintentional, 12.5 percent are due to suicide, and the remaining 6 percent are undetermined (2013).

Of the 2.5 million ER visits annually from drug misuse and abuse, *1.4 million of these were related to pharmaceuticals*, both prescription and over the counter.

10. Health care costs in the USA due to use of tobacco is an estimated $130 billion, alcohol $25 billion, illicit drugs $11 billion, and $700 billion in costs related to crime, lost work productivity and accidents annually.

Despite these alarming statistics, we continue to advertise, prescribe, and consume killer substances; we perform and undergo extensive surgeries and push strong pharmaceuticals all in the name of "crisis medicine" while ignoring the logic and benefits of preventive medicine.[‡]

The third challenge involves the way we choose and train our medical personnel. Book sense, rote memorization, and test-taking skills are highlighted, while basic common sense and communication skills are often overlooked. Technological diagnosis, treatment, electronic records, and rapid precise billing are all well and good, but the time and effort spent on basic patient care is shortened. Such is the case of the creation of "superbugs." The cultural norm is that of over-prescribing as a means of "coverage" or pro-

---

[‡] National Institute on Drug Abuse (NIDA), Trends and Statistics, National Survey on Drug Use and Health (NS-DUH) (2014).

tection. Infants/children are given multiple doses of antibiotics while in the hospital nursery, the ER, and again in the pediatrician's office. Adults take huge amounts of antibiotics and even steroids for head colds, sinusitis, flu, and rhinitis, which are unrelated to their viral causes, but as "coverage" for possible accompanying bacteria. This practice often leads to the inability of the immune system to develop, maintain equilibrium, and function properly. Such protocols are known to be excessive, yet we express alarm when there are increasing cases of drug-resistant / AMR (antimicrobial resistance) superbugs dominating hospitals and clinics. Not only does the overuse of antibiotics cause mutations in the bacteria and viruses, but there is also a huge disruption in the effectivity of the immunity of the population.

At least two million people become infected with antibiotic resistant bacteria and twenty-three thousand die as a direct result. Protection and prevention are of utmost importance. First, do not take antibiotics that were not explicitly prescribed by your doctor. Do not demand antibiotics of your doctor unless it is indicated. Do not take antibiotics that were not prescribed to you for your specific illness. A good 25 percent of colds and flu are viral in nature and not amenable to antibiotics. Implement common basic hygienic methods to contain disease and prevent its spread, like avoiding touching much used surfaces, washing hands thoroughly and often, and avoiding eating uncooked meat. If you must take antibiotics, they should be clearly labelled and appropriately dosed. Physicians and patients should share as complete an understanding about the condition and treatment as possible given the circumstances.[§]

USA health statistics give it a ranking of seventeenth worldwide, i.e. of seventeen industrialized/developed nations. This is unacceptable and is due to the following:

1. Failure to provide health care to all (poverty generates illness)

2. Failure to reduce costs (poverty generates illness)

3. Failure to institute preventive measures (entire population generates illness)

USA Health Care System ranks thirty-seventh worldwide. USA statistics of disease, disability, and death are far higher in the population without private health insurance than the population that is covered. The USA is the *only* developed nation that does not provide all its citizens with equitable, universally available health care.

---

§   Antibiotic Resistance Threats in the Unites States, 2013: CDC report.

Our insurance system is defective as it will pay for expensive surgery but not for prevention of that very surgery in the first place. For example, a quadruple bypass patient is celebrated as a hero for surviving the surgery instead of the person who remains healthy and has no surgery. Nothing is said or done about the lifestyle choices that the patient made that caused the coronary blockage in the first place.¶

The fourth challenge to American healthcare lies in the nature of our health care delivery: the principle and practice of treatment AFTER the disease is firmly established. This inadequate principle will endure as long as a for-profit system remains in place. The parade of sick people seeking miracle cures after the onset and firm hold of disease conditions will be continuous.

The following are a few case examples to illustrate the points. TW are the initials of a 65 year old hypertensive man who quit smoking five years prior to his triple bypass heart surgery. A proud and frequent displayer of his surgical scar and astronomical hospital bill, he never mentions the outrageously fatty diet he enjoyed before becoming a "cardiac patient."

SR is a morbidly obese type 2 diabetic, who suffers terribly with the pain and debilitation of fibromyalgia. She takes an oral hypoglycemic medication as well as unusually large amounts of painkillers and antidepressants and seldom

---

¶ From the National Center for Health Statistics: 2014 World Health Organization (WHO).

has normal blood sugar levels upon testing. She longs for relief while continuing to gulp down sugary drinks, high-calorie snacks, and eat starchy entrees on a daily basis.

BR is a sixty-year-old female chain-smoker with tender lymph nodes and a diagnosis of esophageal cancer for which she underwent surgery and current radiation therapy. She complains of nausea and morning sickness and demands stronger painkillers.

DT carries diagnoses of both lupus and Hodgkin's lymphoma with a severely dysfunctional immune system and a history of multiple doses of antihistamines and antibiotics for frequent sinusitis, rhinitis, and bronchitis. She just started a course on methotrexate, cyclophosphamide, and cis-dichlorodiammineplatinum (cis-platinum).**

JG is a sixty-eight-year-old postmenopausal, hypertensive, overweight lady, with persistent arthritis unresponsive to anti-inflammation medications but tolerable on painkillers. She constantly renews the prescriptions that she regards as the most important part of her daily existence.

EF is a seventy-five-year-old hypertensive arthritic diabetic lady who carries her thirteen medications in a bag attached to her walker. She takes Tramadol (50mg), Vicodin ES (7.5mg), and Gabapentin (300mg) for pain,

---

**   Cis-Dichlorodiammineplatinum: combination chemotherapy and cross-resistance studies with tumors in mice. Schabel FM Jr, et al Cancer Treatment Reports (1979, 63 (9–10):1459–1473)).

Meloxicam (7.5mg), and Nabumetone (500mg) for osteoarthritis, Zoloft for depression, Valium for anxiety, Prilosec for heartburn, Metoprolol (25mg), and Hyzaar (50mg) for hypertension, aspirin (81mg) for heart condition, Brimonidine and Latanoprost eyedrops for glaucoma and Metformin twice a day to control her blood sugar. She cannot feel the soles of her feet and has difficulty forming a complete sentence.

It doesn't have to be that way.

Possible solutions to unhealthy problems:

TW needs to stop boasting about his scar tissue and pay attention to his diet, weight, and degree of physical activity. He needs heart-healthy foods that improve his blood circulation and reduce his risk of further coronary artery damage.

SR needs to lose the weight, stop the sodas, eat a balanced diet of low glycemic foods, good fats, and plant-based proteins, and indulge in a regimen of regular exercise.

BR needs to stop smoking cigarettes completely and adopt a strict diet of anticancer foods, botanicals, and supplements. A decisive increase in physical activity, stress-control breathing techniques, and positive mental enforcement of healing would be of utmost benefit when compared to the results and complications offered by painkillers.

DT would benefit from a consultation with an integrative medicine specialist in oncology who may help with the addition of dietary, exercise, stress reduction, mental and spiritual stabilization, and positive reinforcement strategies to maximize her results.

JG must lose the excess weight through strategies designed for her specific situation. Natural control mechanisms for inflammation reduction that target the cause are far more effective than painkillers and anti-inflammation medications, and without the side effects.

EF needs a complete reevaluation of her medication regimen. Replacing some of the more potent doses with lifestyle modifications would benefit her tremendously.

Disease prevention before *it becomes established makes much more sense than treatment after the fact.*

Possible solutions to political and business influence on health care:

A health care system in which everyone is covered under a universal single payer, which includes "preventive care" as a primary discipline would reduce costs by improving administrative efficiency, reducing the number of "encounters," establish earlier diagnoses, and lead to more effective treatments.

The health care system would be rewarded for a healthy population (instead of large agribusiness, for-profit hospital conglomerates, and parasitic insurance corporations) by having manageable budgets and prevention of catastrophic debts to patients.

Health covering live births, deaths, disease prevalence, expenditures per capita, and total expenditures per percentage of GDP for all the industrialized countries in which universal health care is available are better than those of the United States. There is less prevalence of disease and lower expenditure on health care in the population that is covered by preventive health care. We need to implement some of these strategies and get insurance and for profit businesses out of health care.[††]

Possible solutions to the stagnation of medical care:

The way we treat disease has changed over the last one hundred years: from art, science and tradition, to a heavy reliance on science, and almost total neglect of tradition or art. Despite huge advances in technology, such as CAT and MRI and intricate laser and trauma repair procedures, chronic diseases are more prevalent than ever before even when adjusted for advancements on age. Suppose we focus on the health of individuals, communities, populations with the goal being to promote health, protection against and prevent disease, disability, and premature death. If measures and techniques in medical practice were directed more toward disease prevention rather than disease treatment, our results would improve tremendously. By including "all the other options available" to recognize the threat or possibility of disease and beginning measures to

††   WHO: Global Health Observatory data repository.

block the onset of said disease, healthcare would be much more successful than it is now.

The whole individual should be identified and assessed, with complex links and associations to personal and social connections that play a role in development and progression of disease, before he or she becomes a statistical patient. If the typical patient has metabolic syndrome with high blood sugar, high blood pressure, obesity, and high cholesterol that leads to heart disease, stroke, and diabetes with possible blindness, loss of limbs, debilitating vascular system, and premature death, all strongly linked to inflammation, poor immunity, and unhealthy lifestyle habits, why not identify the possibilities and probabilities and take measures to implement strategies to control the physiological parameters and avoid the disease?

The goal is to achieve and maintain natural health and well-being, through integrative medicine techniques of Andrew Weil, MD, director of integrative medicine at the University of Arizona, Tucson, that include a complete range of options for disease prevention and treatment.

Natural health practices (like drinking medicinal teas and eating organic food) offer protective measures by boosting immunity and inhibiting drug-resistant bugs. It must be understood that natural products do not have the same acute medicinal effects as pharmaceutical drugs. They are not fast-acting or as potent in effect. They do not repair severely damaged tissue and organ systems. They are not intended to counteract acute trauma or reverse serious infection in a matter of a few doses. However, when taken regularly, they do help prevent the onset and progression of many chronic diseases. It should also be noted that natural products are not regulated by government agencies and therefore may be "fake" or ineffective as well.

Traditional medicine practices aim to keep people well. Plant defense mechanisms take the threat of microbial and immunological diseases and create phytochemicals to block or inhibit them. Humans and other animals benefit greatly from these transactions: foxglove to digitalis for heart disease, cinchona bark to quinine for malaria, willow bark to salicylic acid (aspirin) for inflammation and pain, penicillin molds to antibiotics for septic infections, and curare for anesthesia. Natural botanicals are used externally and internally, are inexpensive, and have a low rate of toxicity. Pharmaceuticals, especially for chronic diseases, are potent, fast-acting, expensive, and in most cases, do not provide a cure, so must be purchased over and over again to soothe recurring symptoms. Identifying and addressing the cause of disease would have much more satisfying and effective results.

While large investments in the advanced technology to remove and destroy cancerous tumors is heroic and fantastic, when it works, why not prevent the tumors in the first place...through similar expenditures in natural health.

Prevention is easier and more effective than treatment.

We, as physicians, need to address the underlying problems of poor health, the inadequate diet, and lifestyle factors that cause or contribute to the disease in the first place. Then use preventive measures or treat accordingly and specifically.

The human body has the innate ability to heal itself. DNA repair mechanisms with antioxidant enhancement are readily available in healthy cells. Learning to understand one's own body signals can give positive reinforcement to improve and maintain health. Go beyond "there is nothing more we can do for you." Address the cause of the problem; do not just cover it over with medications.

Coping with chronic illness begins with preventive measures and the goal of preventive medicine is to achieve maximum healing with minimum intervention.

1

Causes of Diseases

Once you identify the causes of diseases, in many cases, they can be prevented. Many adverse conditions and diseases are the result of a breakdown in body systems due to diet and lifestyle choices and can, therefore, often be prevented or even reversed if treated early and properly.

—A. L. Anduze, MD

Good health saves billions of dollars in capital, immense expenditures of energy, and unnecessary stress. So why not invest it in preventive measures instead of after-the-fact expensive pharmaceuticals and complicated procedures? We are all susceptible to disease, whether it be due to indulgences of the affluent or afflictions of the poor. How we respond to the exposure and/or deficiency determines the course and outcome.

Disease Susceptibility

Genetic factors related to genotype activity and phenotype expression in combination with environmental factors and lifestyle choices are responsible for a large portion of human diseases. (1) Genetic markers are turned on or off depending on either chance or a mutation induced by internal or external signaling. For example, the markers of Alzheimer's disease may be present in an individual, but they must be turned on to be expressed as dementia. Likewise, markers of rheumatoid arthritis, type 2 diabetes, glaucoma, and breast cancer can be influenced by lifestyle choices based on diet, stress levels, external toxins, and internal hormonal reactions. (2) In addition to the expected defects from environment and interbreeding within the social and hereditary structure, genes can be triggered by diet-related substances like sugar, gluten, lactose, and salt. Environmental stress factors like toxin exposure to substances such as plastics, aluminum, mercury, polychlorinated biphenyls (PCB), glyphosates (in weed killers), and secondhand smoke can induce mutations which contribute to neurological conditions like multiple sclerosis (MS), autism , amyotropic lateral sclerosis (ALS), and various cancers.

Some diseases, like hypertension, heart disease, diabetes, and some cancers are more prevalent and carry higher morbidity and mortality rates in individuals of certain ethnicities. Genetically linked diseases like sickle-cell anemia and distinct syndromes are related to the genotypic composition of the individual. As "race" *is a social concept and does not in itself cause disease, I feel it is not appropriate to constantly refer to it in scientific matters. All humans are of the same race—homo sapiens. Any variations in physical reactions to disease are due more to the influences of individual behavior, culture, economic status, and access to quality health care than to innate DNA differences between "the races."* "Minorities" is another term used that denotes some kind of inferiority and high susceptibility to disease, when in fact it is lack of access to early health care and inadequate health insurance that is responsible for a large part of the morbidity seen. In the USA, the term "black" is used to denote a specific group of people of color and high rates of obesity, diabetes, colorectal cancer, hypertension, glaucoma, and heart disease are attributed to the group as a whole. However, within that group are individuals with DNA that ranges from 95 percent Caucasian to 5 percent African. The high incidence and prevalence of these diseases in the population of color should instead be reviewed in terms of exposure and reaction to stress. The high incidence of vision-threatening glaucoma and hypertension in young, black males is directly related to high levels of emotional and environmental stress. The high level of alcoholism in Native Americans may be due in part to a genetic propensity, but the obesity, poor nutrition, and poor health are the basis for the high mortality.

Immune System Compromise

Most preventable diseases are caused by or associated with a weak immune system.

Elements of a strong immune system can block the diabetic genes from being expressed by low exposure to sugar and starches. Similarly, alcoholism, cancer, chronic depression, and arthritis genes can be adequately suppressed. Immuno-incompetence leaves the system open to attack and direct damage as well as internal dysfunction. Pathogens, which may be organisms or toxins, can damage the host directly, overwhelm its immune system, or cause the latter to damage its own tissues, giving rise to autoimmune diseases. Immune cells infiltrate every body system and have a role in every disease occurrence. The immune system is regulated by hormones. Toxins disrupt the hormonal balance and cause disease. Ageing has its own characteristic response to disease challenge, in that the very young and very old are particularly susceptible to disease. This susceptibility is due to the presence of an immature immune system on the one hand and the decline in tissue maintenance and repair capacities on the other. A weak immune system with inadequate numbers or poor quality T and B cells can allow disease to flourish in the body. A strong immune system with a healthy and adequate population of functional cells can combat disease better than a weak system with decreased numbers or dysfunctional cells, which result from a combination of genetics, environment and lifestyle choices.

All the strategies of natural health are associated with and rely heavily on a functional immune system.

Inflammation

Almost all disease conditions are associated with some form of inflammation, the cellular response to local injury of redness, swelling, and pain, which derives from both a good and a bad immune system. A good system responds to an attack with a measured issue of T and B cells and their metabolites that heal and repair. A bad system responds erratically and irregularly to provide an overreaction or an underreaction that results in crippling inflammation. When the response is chronic and can result in lingering conditions like arthritis, enteritis, bronchitis, neuropathies, and neurodegenerations.

The medical school mnemonic VINDICATE is one way to reference the causes of disease, each of which involves some form of inflammation though from different sources. **v**ascular, **i**nfection (inflammation), **n**eoplasm (cancer), **d**rugs (toxins), **i**ntervention (iatrogenic), **c**ongenital (genetic), **a**utoimmune, **t**rauma, **e**ndocrine (metabolic) are mainly associated with poor general internal health and some external environmental exposures. An "S" should be added to make it vindicates, as **s**tress plays a major role in the onset and prevalence of most of these diseases. Because such a large number of patients suffer from a combination of several of these disease processes, it should be termed *"total body inflammation."*

Stress is one of the most important risk factors in the cause of disease. In times of emotional and physical stress, the adrenal glands release excess cortisol, the "inflammation hormone." At normal levels, it is produced from cholesterol stores in response to physical exercise, routine bodily functions, and acute stress, with beneficial results. In excess, such as that resulting from chronic stress it results in the onset and progression of damages to every cell, tissue, and organ system through the inflammation response. Mental imbalances, forms of depression, and psycho-spiritual losses can lead to profound cortisol-related disease complexes like cancer, endocrine diseases, autoimmune disorders, and heart disease. Situations in which stress is chronic, such stress wears down the body and the mind, resulting in damage to all systems.

Research suggests that daily stressors are major factors in the poor health status of a large segment of the population in the United States. The daily stress that is encountered, absorbed, and resisted is directly related to the biochemical and physiological factors that are associated with hypertension, stroke, type 2 diabetes, obesity, central nervous system disorders, and inflammatory diseases. A significant reduction in the level of stress that an individual incurs and internalizes is a key factor in the prevention of many diseases. Stress reduction can be achieved through strategies like avoidance of stressors, social support, individual dietary adjustments, and self-awareness. Having a solid social circle of family and friends on which to rely in times of stress is an incredibly effective factor in stress control. Just having someone close to say that "everything will be all right" and "I will help" is sometimes all the medicine that is needed. Avoiding the urge to overeat to satisfy emotional upset is right up there with social support. Remaining calm and fully aware of the circumstances that lead to the stressful situation can more often lead to a successful outcome, than a total collapse.[3, 4, 5]

Poor Dietary Practices

Diet influences health more than weight.

The ability to repair, rebuild, and regenerate cells of all systems depends on intake of essential nutrients which in turn influence hormonal balance. Especially in the USA, we overconsume industrialized, processed food with little to no nutritional value: processed sugars (carbohydrates), fat-laden grains, and foods altered by fermentation, freezing, dehydrating, and questionable germination. Some processed foods start out as natural plants, which are then stripped of their natural phytochemicals, fibers, vitamins, and minerals to isolate a single ingredient that gives a desired effect. Then additives, flavorings, colorings, preservatives, and packaging, all chemicals, are added to the product. Livestock, poultry, and even hatchlings are injected with hormones to increase the frequency of pregnancies and enable rapid growth, which will suppress or stimulate the consumers' own hormones and body systems in an unnatural way. Some 85 percent of our annually prescribed antibiotics are fed to livestock to prevent infection and stimulate growth.

Contemporary food does not contain the same levels of vitamin and mineral contents than prior to the advent of supermarkets and the industrialization of the food supply in the 1940s. Even natural unprocessed food is of lower quality due to production in poor-grade soil laden with chemical fertilizers and pesticides designed to give higher yields. So even most fruits and vegetables, unless they are organically grown, are loaded with toxins. Two bad things happen here—the effects of the toxicity of the chemicals on our organ systems, and the fact that our produce cannot produce the antioxidant level of phytochemicals that would be effective against carriers of disease. Both mineral and vitamin uptake from the soil is compromised. Improper diet and poor elimination allow cumulative tissue damages by toxins. In addition, chronic dehydration due to inadequate intake of pure clean water contributes hugely to the consequences of poor health. Dehydration is associated with seizures, low blood pressure, kidney failure, medication ineffectiveness, interference with basic digestion of nutrients and elimination of toxins.[6]

Eat organic and local whenever possible.

Poor Lifestyle Choices

In the 1950s, shortly after the food industrialization era, the sedentary lifestyle arrived where TV dinners and packaged food became the societal norm. One could live quite comfortably devoid of social contact, or mental stimulation, with poor dietary practices, bad habits (such as smoking cigarettes), high alcohol intake, psychoactive drugs, lack of sleep, and unsafe sexual practices with potential STD exposure. This was the time when it became all too convenient for one's lifestyle choices to take a downturn; consequentially, the health of the general public plunged along with it. Today we live in an environment that is toxic, we add more toxins to our bodies by consuming artificial food, and our cortisol levels due to stress are higher than ever.[7]

Environmental Toxicity

The risk of contracting diseases greatly increases with exposure to environmental toxins and drugs.

The human body can keep all systems in balance. But when it is influenced by foreign substances, the balance, or homeostasis, is disrupted. Though one may believe one is functioning at optimum capacity, it is important to observe the validity of such claims when the average household environment is riddled with toxicity. The typical urban setting is rife with plastics (BPA), and synthetic chemicals like PCBs (polychlorinated biphenyls), fertilizers, and pesticides with glyphosates (many of which are associated with autism and hormone disruptive neonatal developmental defects). Toxins are present in food as additives and other processing chemicals, as well as home structures, furniture, lawns, and along sidewalks and stores and workplaces. There are pollutants from cars, trucks, and factories, which make up the bulk of our vast industrial system. Toxins like aluminum products and anticholinergic drugs may cause a breakdown of the blood-brain barrier (capillary system that carries nutrients and removes wastes to and from the brain tissues), which results in leakage throughout the neuronal system thus leading to cellular dysfunction associated with dementia, autism, Parkinson's, and ALS. (Be careful of cooking at too frequently using aluminum foil at high heat.) The effects of cell phone use and exposure to high tech electronics in the form of frequency sensitivity have been duly noted, but have yet to be fully studied. Add to this, the ubiquitous stress factors of daily living and the human body is open to the onset and establishment of diseases of all kinds.

Trauma/Injury

Traumatic injuries also leave the body in a state of vulnerability to infection and disrepair. Iatrogenic interventions with surgeries and medications may lead to other systems' breakdowns. For everything introduced into the body, there is a reaction, a change, and the body "pays "a price whether it is good or bad.

Lack of Exercise

Inactivity leads to immune system dysfunction and lapses in all other organ systems, often resulting in obesity, which further compounds poor circulation (vascularity) leading to chronic low-grade inflammation. This is a prominent feature of arthritis, diabetes, hypertension, and dementia.

Active overweight is better than inactive normal weight.

Traditional Medicine

Placebo effects exist in both science and the arts. In medicine, these are healing responses loosely based on expectations, which may be activated by mind-mediated mechanisms with a real scientific basis in brain activity. They exist, and they work. In some traditional cultures, the cause of disease is attributed to the loss of vital energy and/ or the presence of negative spiritual influences. Prevention and cure are achieved by a combination of physiochemical and mind controlling practices particular to that culture and not left only to the potency of synthetic drugs and extensive surgical procedures.

Prevention: to identify and avert disease before it sets in.

Eating a well-balanced diet of high antioxidant fruits and vegetables, whole grains, seeds, nuts, lean and plant-based proteins, and good fats with lots of omega-3 and 6 fatty acids will lead to an increase in natural killer T cells and B cells, which drive a healthy immune system response.

People who consume a diet rich in carotenoids from natural foods suffer less from chronic diseases than those who are deficient. Optimal health and well being can be achieved and maintained by the reduction in inflammatory disease, cardiovascular disease, onset and progression of cancer through balanced nutrition and attention to physical activity, hydration, and active control/management of blood chemistry (blood glucose, blood pressure, serum lipids) through sanitation, appropriate vaccinations, avoidance of infection, and chemical toxins.

Note that exercise contributes hugely to good health and plays a leading role in almost all forms of disease prevention.

References:

1. Influence of genetics on disease susceptibility and progression. Duff GW, et al. Nutr Rev. 2007.

2. The discovery of human genetic variations and their use as disease markers: past, present and future. Ku CS, et al. J Hum Genet 2010 Jul; 55(7):403–15.

3. Cortisol: Its role in stress, Inflammation, and indications for Diet Therapy. Dina Aronson, MS, RD, Today's Dietician, Vol. 11 No.11, P. 38.

4. Race-Ethnicity, Poverty, Urban Stressors, and Telomere length in a Detroit Community-based sample. Geronimus AT, et al. J Health Soc Behav. 2015.

5. Giving support to others reduces sympathetic nervous system-related responses to stress. Inagaki TK, et al. Psychophysiology. 2015.

6. Mechanisms by which dehydration may lead to chronic kidney disease. Roncal-Jimenez C, et al. Ann Nutr Metab. 2015.

7. High cortisol awakening response is associated with impaired error monitoring and decreased, post-error adjustment. Zhang L, et al. Stress. 2015.

Self-Assessment Questions Concerning Current Health Status[‡‡]

1. How can I live longer and maintain good health into old age?

2. How can I keep my senses of sight and hearing into old age?

3. Can taking pharmaceutical drugs prevent disease?

4. How can I reduce the frequency of doctor visits and keep medical costs down?

5. How can I avoid infectious diseases when travelling in a foreign country?

6. How can I get vitamin D from the sun without getting skin cancer?

[‡‡] See answers in appendix.

7. What foods can I eat to prevent disease? And what foods should I avoid?

8. If my parents had diabetes, hypertension, heart disease, Alzheimer's, and arthritis, will I get them too?

9. How can I prevent dementia?

10. How can I keep my cholesterol down without using strong drugs?

11. How can I lose weight naturally and keep it off?

12. Are taking dietary supplements good or bad?

13. Are using skin health and beauty products okay? What diet is best for skin care?

14. Why do some people survive or even repel a disease exposure while others of the same age and environment succumb?

15. What are the effects of GMO foods on the human body?

16. How can I escape cancer?

17. If I quit smoking, will I still get heart disease?

18. If I quit smoking now, what are the chances that I will start again?

19. How do I just get up and exercise? I can't do it.

20. I'm old. Why doesn't everybody just leave me alone?

21. I live in the city and do not have access to fresh organic food, and when it is available, it is too expensive. How can I avoid toxic foods and pollutants in the air and water?

22. Does omega-3 fish oil really work to improve health?

23. What herbs and spices should I use in the kitchen?

24. I am allergic to everything. Even the drugs they give me to stop allergies make me break out. What can I do?

25. I'm sixty-eight years old, and I can no longer ski the double black diamond trails or surf the biggest waves. What gives here?

2

Six Basic Strategies for Disease Prevention

A healthy immune system and a low level of inflammation are important factors in reducing the risk of developing both acute and chronic diseases. Exercise, nutrition, stress control, social connections, mental stimulation, and avoidance of high-risk behavior are basic strategies that are directed at achieving this goal. The identification of risk factors and early symptoms is essential to implementing prevention measures to stop the onset and progression of these disease conditions. For example, the prevention of type 2 diabetes, hypertension, arthritis, cancer, and heart disease can be realized through a healthy lifestyle using research-proven strategies, natural products, and common sense, rather than strong, sometimes toxic, pharmaceuticals and interventional surgery after the fact.

As aging is a natural and inevitable part of existence so is accompanying disease and disability. As Dan Buettner so aptly illustrates in his *Blue Zones* series, set in areas of the world where longevity is the highest, the rate of aging is influenced by a combination of genetics, environment, diet, culture, and degrees of lifestyle simplicity. Despite what we do or don't do to some effect, the human body ages and eventually ceases to function. We do, however, have a choice as to *how* we age. Since most negative feelings about aging are based on fear, our best choice is a positive outlook. We wish to avoid the pain and dysfunction of arthritis and neurological degenerations, the inconvenience of vision and hearing loss, memory loss of Alzheimer's and dementia, and the life-threatening effects of hypertension, diabetes, and cardiac disease. Though aging cannot be stopped, many physicians are looking beyond Western medicine with its toxic drugs and complicated procedures and toward the traditional practices of prevention and maintenance to enhance the experience and quality of life in the best way possible. Regular checkups are still essential for early diagnosis of common disease conditions, as treatments are more effective when implemented earlier. An integrative medicine approach to easing the journey into old age involves *lifestyle changes* with problem-specific plans for stimulating the mind, preserving the senses and prolonging the quality of life.

Exercise

Exercise, as seen from studies involving communities with high longevity rates, was determined to be the first and most important strategy for good health and disease prevention. Regular physical activity is better at preventing and curing disease than pharmaceutical drugs and complex therapies.

Note that the emphasis is on "regular." The human body is aptly constructed for movement and continued physical activity serves to

1. maintain body tone, balance, and flexibility;

2. control stress hormones (cortisol, epinephrine, norepinephrine);

3. release endorphin hormones (relieves the effects of stress);

4. eliminate toxins through perspiration;

5. improve mood (both anxiety and depression);

6. improve immune system function and reduce inflammation;

7. improve bone mass especially in postmenopausal women;

8. regulate blood sugar by decreasing insulin levels;

9. improve cardiac function, lower blood pressure, and improve blood flow to organs;

10. maintain healthy weight levels;

11. reduce risk of colon cancer;

12. increase oxygen rich blood to the brain (avoids dementia);

13. increase body temperature (relaxes tense muscles).

Increasing the blood flow to the brain by walking is an effective way of reducing the risk of dementia. A daily walk or walking at least three times a week, for a minimum of thirty minutes at a time is recommended by many health providers. Swimming is good for improving breathing, muscle tone, and joint health. Aerobic training helps heart failure patients by enhancing oxygen capacity and blood flow dynamics. Walking regularly reduces the risk of colon cancer by decreasing the time that food stays in the GI tract and reducing the levels of prostaglandins that cause colon inflammation. Free weight training helps develop and maintain bone density to reduce the risk of fractures. Exercise not only strengthens locomotion muscles, but respiratory and cardiac muscles as well. Burning fat calories in the morning and carbohydrates in the evening effectively maintains normal weight. Structured exercises like hatha yoga and tai chi can benefit flexibility and balance.

In general, movement is always better than sedentary. While a reduction in caloric intake can be directed at losing weight, exercise will keep it off.

Goal: increase and improve total body blood circulation, effective cleansing of the lymphatic system, elimination of wastes and toxins.

Recommended physical activity: may be divided into three categories. (1) Aerobic exercises: walking, biking, running, hiking, rowing, and most other "sports" activities that demand oxygen consumption. These benefit the heart, increase red blood cell production, enable weight loss, increase immune system function, and release endorphins, the "feel good" hormones that reduce stress and depression sensitivity. A regular walk or jog for thirty minutes, three times per week, and fifteen minutes activity on alternate days is a good regimen to maintain in the over thirty age group. Do two days activity that breaks a sweat (thirty to sixty minutes) and five days a week regular fifteen-minute activity, which may consist of warm up and cool down stretches, toe touches, hamstring stretch, calf stretch, light weight training, push-ups, sit ups, chin ups, leg lifts, wall sits, biceps curls and a variety of other structured repetitive movements. (2) Anaerobic exercises consist mainly of weight training and strengthening muscle and maintaining bone, joint, and tendon health. This includes resistance machines, bands, and equipment with opposing contractions for increasing muscle size and endurance. (3) Flexibility and balance exercises include stretching, yoga, tai chi, and martial arts movements that involve coordination of the body and the mind to increase muscle tone and extend range.

It is just as important to enlist the advice of an educated trainer before beginning an exercise regimen as it is to consult your physician concerning you're the status of your health.

> Walking is a man's best medicine.
>
> —Hippocrates

Nutrition and Diet

Let food be thy medicine and medicine be thy food.

—Hippocrates

Proper diet and nutrition remain at the forefront of healthy aging strategies.

A balance of protein, carbohydrates, and fats, antioxidants for control of inflammation and a strong immune system, timely elimination and detoxification, as well as stress and weight control, are the goals to be achieved for optimum health. The "modern health promoting diet" (MHPD) is high in vegetables, fruits, whole grains, legumes, nuts, and seeds and low in calories. The essential vitamins are C, A, E, B complex, lutein, selenium, magnesium, zinc and omega-3 fatty acids, which are found in cold-water fish, flaxseed oil, nuts, garlic, broccoli, soy, beans, citrus fruits, and melons. When unable to obtain fresh food, supplements, though never as effective as whole food, may be used. A daily multivitamin should contain most of the above vitamins and minerals. However, it is advised that one take a multivitamin that is specific to their sex and age group.

The quantity of food intake is just as important as the content. A reduction in the amount of red meat consumption as well as portion size of each food group to the amount that will fit into the palm of your hand will further enhance positive nutrition without the tendency to overeat.

Since the quality of our commercially prepared food is not what it should be, attention must be paid to the acquisition of health promoting foods whenever possible. The following is a brief list of appropriate vitamins, minerals, and supplements that can help in maintaining good health.

1.   Cholesterol control: oatmeal, bran cereals, lecithin, Vitamins B3 and B6, red yeast rice

2.   Stress control: folic acid or folates, calcium and magnesium, garlic , ashwagandha

3.   Vision support: ginkgo biloba and cayenne for retinal circulation; bilberry, eyebright and lutein for macula integrity and function

4.   Prostate function: saw palmetto, pumpkin seeds, pygeum, zinc, and nettles

5.   Joint and bone repair: glucosamine and chondroitin, SAMe and MSM

6.   Excess blood clotting and stroke prevention: garlic, ginger, and aspirin (blood thinners)

7.   Inflammation control: antioxidants like green, black and jasmine tea, red wine, dark chocolate, ginger, and turmeric

8.   Liver protection: milk thistle, artichoke, shiitake mushrooms

9.   Heart function: coenzyme Q10, garlic, omega 3 fish oils

10. Degenerative diseases: Reischi mushrooms, Rhodiola rosea, Cordyceps

Hydration: Most importantly, daily *water* intake of one-half your body weight in ounces for the average-sized individual potentiates all general nutrition. Water burns fat, suppresses hunger, renews skin turgor, and saves all organs from deterioration.

Table 1

Good food that promotes the prevention and reduction of inflammation:

Omega-3 fatty acids (cold-water fish oil ,flaxseed, walnuts), antioxidants (vitamins A, C, E, B complex, folic acid) Extra virgin olive oil , organic canola oil Garlic, ginger, onions Green tea Whole foods (fruit and vegetables) Fiber (wheat with kernels) Turmeric Plant proteins, mushrooms, mustard Berries, nuts, seeds Honey, stevia, agave (natural sweeteners) Water Soybeans.[§§]

[§§]   Soybeans in the USA are mostly GMO and, as such, is not naturally grown but rather genetically composed or engineered in addition to being sprayed with pesticides. Excessive quantities may lower testosterone levels in men and may contribute to hormonal imbalance in women. As of this writing, its consumption should be limited.

Basic Cooking Recommendations

Try not to cook on an empty stomach. Too much "tasting" can and will add unnecessary calories. Avoid adding too much salt (one teaspoon is enough for most recipes) or too much oil (one tablespoon of olive oil is about 120 calories).

Table 2

Bad foods that promote and sustain inflammation:

High fructose corn syrup (HFCS) *in most packaged/ processed foods and drinks* omega 6 fatty acids[¶¶] *(low saturated vegetable oils, sunflower seeds, pecan nuts)* Refined white sugar, white rice Saturated fats/ commercially baked goods, cookies, cakes, pastries Hydrogenated fats/ margarine/ trans fats (doughnuts, coffee cake, buns, biscuits) Chips, fries (*acrylamide*), popcorn Polyunsaturated fats (corn, safflower, coconut oils) Sodas (*refined sugar, artificial sweetener, sulfites*), energy drinks, diet drinks Animal protein (*growth hormones, antibiotics*) Wheat (*processed, glutens*) Ketchup (*artificial sweeteners, high fructose corn syrup (HFCS)*) Hot dogs, luncheon meats (*sodium nitrite is a known carcinogen*)

¶¶   It should be noted that omega-6 foods, like pork sausage, cheddar cheese, and eggs fried in vegetable oil, corn chips, commercially baked cookies, candies, and cakes, should be consumed only in limited amounts and in conjunction with omega-3 foods. A healthy ratio is 1:4. Simply adhering to this chart will improve or maintain your health tremendously.

Canned soup (*monosodium glutamate (*MSG)) New canned soup (disodium glythalamate (DSG))

When ingested on a daily basis, any one or all of these "bad" foods can increase the risk of heart disease, stroke, diabetes, hypertension, and cancer.

Elimination and detoxification must be regular. Prune juice is very effective. Psyllium and/or flaxseed in a powdered form are available to purchase organic, convenient, and moderately priced. A home-made mixture of apple cider vinegar, extra virgin olive oil, and lemon (one teaspoon each) is excellent when ingested on a weekly basis. Try to eat a*ge-appropriate* food. Most red meats are indigestible at age seventy and sodas with high sugar at age eighty are a sure means of triggering or aggravating diabetes. Avoid foods and vitamins that promise to cure. Beware of the effects of medications. Aside from their high incidence of toxicity and side effects, there is a definitive effect on basic sense of taste. Read the labels of all you ingest or use on your body. Ask questions and follow instructions in order to avoid disease occurrences, treatment failures, and poor outcomes.

Basic Dietary and Nutritional Recommendations

Eat organic when you can. Eat foods that are local, seasonal, and appropriate to the region in which you live. Both plants and animals consumed by humans contain nutritional value and offer mechanisms for immune defense based on the region in which they are found. Coca leaf and maca root greatly enhance stamina and endurance at high altitudes in the Andes mountains, rhodiola rosea and eleuthero root guard against the stresses of extreme cold and nutritional deficiencies of the Arctic regions, and fruits high in vitamin C and energy supplying sugars are abundant in the Tropics. Plant-based foods prevent diseases like type 2 diabetes, heart disease, hypertension, and cancer. Foods lose their nutritional value when there is long period between the time they were picked or harvested and put on the table. Foods that have been subjected to artificial fertilization, pesticides, or added chemicals needed to give them a long shelf life, do not have the same quality are fresh natural products. For the average person, protein should constitute 30 percent, carbohydrates, 40 percent, and good fats, 30 percent of the diet. Dietary portions should vary by age and level of activity. An older sedentary person would eat less protein, more carbohydrates in the form of vegetables and fruit, than a younger, more active person. The portion size should be the amount of each food group that fits in the palm of your hand. The nutrition level and vitamin and mineral intake should be commensurate with your age and activity levels. The total intake should be equal to the output in energy expended.

Four small meals a day evenly spaced are recommended for good digestion, absorption, and elimination. Reducing the intake of pro-inflammatory foods and increasing anti-inflammatory foods will promote good health.

A modified balanced diet of protein, fats, and carbohydrates is better than one that concentrates on only one food group—i.e., vegetables.

Obesity, a number one target of disease prevention, is strongly associated with heart disease, hypertension, diabetes, stroke, and cancer. Avoid crash diets and eat sensibly to achieve and maintain optimal weight.

Table 3

Suggested Nutritional Formula for Natural Health and Disease Prevention

Multivitamin (age appropriate multivitamin)

Garlic (one clove raw or chopped cooked; daily)

Berries, nuts, seeds (one handful of either or more; daily)

Vegetables (broccoli, spinach, kale, cauliflower, mushrooms; four servings of either daily)

Legumes (lentils, beans; one cup)

Moringa leaves (in salad, stew, over eggs, raw; one teaspoon biweekly)

Whole grains (brown rice, quinoa, 1 cup; four grams daily)

Wheat germ (one cup; biweekly)

Anticancer tea (green tea, anamú, lemongrass, graviola; one cup of each or either, biweekly)

Turmeric (powder or raw; one teaspoon daily in food, tea, or capsule)

Omega 3 (coldwater fish, flaxseed milled or oil, extra virgin olive oil; 1000mg biweekly)

Detoxification (lemon, olive oil, apple cider vinegar mix; one teaspoon, three times a day, once a week)

Water should be an average of eight to ten glasses daily; one-half of one's body weight in ounces

For example, a 140-pound person should drink seventy ounces water = nine glasses or *eight ounces each* daily;

A 180-pound person should drink ninety ounces = eleven glasses daily

Stress Management

> Every stress leaves an indelible scar, and the organism pays for its survival after a stressful situation by becoming a little older.
>
> —Hans Selye (1907–1982)

Under acute stress, the sympathetic nervous system releases the hormones epinephrine and norepinephrine and the hypothalamic-pituitary-adrenal (HPA) system releases glucocorticoids mostly in the form of cortisol. This leads to overuse of energy (*glucocorticoids*) without adequate replacement of basic elements. Too much cortisol in the blood is toxic to many organ cells. Release of free radicals (*oxidative stress*) cause injury to DNA, proteins, and cell membranes. When the parasympathetic nervous system shuts down, the healing process and access to energy reserves become nonfunctional. Decreased energy at the cellular level results in a dysfunctional immune system leaving the body vulnerable to disease.

With chronic stress the release of epinephrine and cortisol is repetitive and prolonged. The damage to tissues and organ systems is slower but, in some cases, more profound. Here emotional stress is more common and is found as a " personal disease" in a societal construct that invites and revels in competition where there is social approval for those who "make it" and punishment in the form of social disapproval for those who don't. Those whom society deems "losers" often become scared, hopeless, and lost—a state that often leads to frustration and illness in the form of anxiety and/or depression.

Physical stress is incurred upon exposure to environmental toxins, pollutants, bad food, and trauma. Similarly, oxidative free radicals, those highly reactive unbalanced molecules are released, which cause severe damage to cells, tissues, and organ systems. Symptoms of physical stress include unexplained weight loss, frequent neck and head pain, decreased appetite, heart palpitations, insomnia, heartburn, and anxiety. There are five basic factors involved in coping with stress: take in a high-energy diet, ensure physical and mental fitness, secure a good social network, get adequate sleep, and keep a calm, restful mind. Good relaxation techniques including breathing exercises, coping mechanisms like journaling, and increased exercise to release good hormones like endorphins will help greatly with stress control. Surround yourself with love. Laughing long, hard and often is medicinal. Aging signs remind us of our mortality and may be a stimulus for spiritual awakening and positive growth. Most importantly, your attitude to the aging process should be one of acceptance and understanding, such that the wisdom that accompanies the later years can best be processed and dispensed. Many things improve with age, not only wine, cheese, and violins, but people too.

There are several natural healthy tonics known as "adaptogens" that are commonly used in northern Europe and parts of Asia to help alleviate stress-related processes. They are highly effective and will be introduced and discussed in chapter 4 in the stress protocol.

Mental Stimulation

Mental stimulation is necessary to avoid dementia and other late onset central nervous system disorders. Continued learning through reading, word puzzles, memory games, and challenging games, exercises the brain cells and circuitry. Traveling to places you've never been before, learning a new language, and enjoying simple things like a walk in the garden or the park all can stimulate brain cells. Pets, hobbies, plants, books, keepsakes are all stimulating, enjoyable, and health-promoting for the brain. They all serve to relieve stress and provide relaxation. Consider meditation with or without yoga, self-guided imagery, music, and expressive art therapy as forms of approaching creative relaxation.

Stresses varying in intensity over a long period of time can lead to brain inflammation and dysfunction of vital neurons. Adequate rest and relaxation are essential for the basic functioning and regeneration of glial cells, which are tasked with the maintenance of neurons and regulation of neurological processes.

A good sleep ensures healthy biorhythms. Basic physiology and metabolism rely on healthy, well-rested cells in order to function. Taking strong, sedative-hypnotic drugs for sleep, like Zolpidem, Halcyon, Ambien, and/or Diazepam suppresses the nervous system, leaves the user impaired, and needing more and more to achieve the same end. Try using natural products like mixtures of melatonin, valerian, chamomile, passionflower, lavender, and hops to achieve adequate rest along with good regulation of biorhythms without the tolerance and chances of addiction. Using mind-body relaxation techniques such as breathing exercise can also achieve substantial brain relaxation.

Social Connections

Social connections, especially healthy relationships with family and friends, are very important for maintaining the sharpness of the mind and avoiding the steep decline into dementia. Regular communication stimulates the mind and provides security in knowing that someone is close at hand when the need arises. Coping with life-changing events such as retirement, feelings of uselessness, loss of a loved one, and changes in living arrangements are very important. Reassurance of some control over one's life activities in the face of loss of independence in transportation and financial responsibilities is helpful. Maintenance of some intimacy with another person or persons and avoidance of mistreatment are also necessary ingredients of social connectivity. Support and pursuit of special interests with like-minded individuals is of utmost importance. Avoid loneliness, stay involved. Simply sharing a meal with others prolongs the event, which in turn improves digestion. Planning and doing are almost equivalent and serve in looking forward with positive anticipation rather than stagnating in dismal dread. Religious organizations also serve as forums to bring people together. Practice open-mindedness and do community service work whenever possible.

Avoidance of High-Risk Behavior

Avoidance of high-risk behavior is self-explanatory.

Nutritional toxins exposure: Stop the intake of bad food (fast food fried in vegetable oils, trans fats, high-glycemic index foods with MSG, aspartame and HFCS), bad habits like smoking cigarettes, excess caffeine, carbonated drinks, excess sugar, illicit drugs, and excessive alcohol intake. Be aware of heavy metals in food and water like methylmercury contamination in fish. Do not cook food in microwave no matter how "safe" they say it is. Radiation always leaks. But if you must use this appliance, use wax paper to cover the container and stand a minimum of eight feet away from the microwave oven when reheating or warming food. When cooking foods on a gas or electric standard oven, use parchment paper to cover the food, then add the aluminum foil to that cover so it has no direct contact with the food.

Environmental Toxins Exposure

Land: Pollutants such as fertilizers with synthetic chemicals, pesticides with DDT and PCB that were banned in the 1960s but are still found in the soil act directly on neural pathways, and glyphosate (weed-killer) residues act directly on gut bacteria to reduce absorption of nutrients and disrupt digestion. Testing of farm families for pesticide in the urine reveal levels below the EPA reference dose of three milligram/kilogram per day, but caution is expressed to minimize exposure nonetheless. Look at who is funding the studies.***#

Air: Chemicals used in the gas and oil industries, like benzene, xylene, toluene, and ethylbenzene move freely in the air and can disrupt the endocrine signaling

***# Glyphosate biomonitoring for farmers and their families: results from Farm Family Exposure Study. Acquavella JF, et al. Environ Health Perspect. 2004.

systems, leading to reproductive, respiratory, and heart conditions. These chemicals are also found in household cleansers, adhesives, detergents, dyes, degreasers, pesticides, polishes, solvents, and paints together with volatile organic compounds (VOC). Sulfur dioxide, nitrogen oxide, lead, and particulate matter are especially prevalent in the urban setting. They cause poor air quality both indoors and outside. It should be noted that the largest carbon dioxide pollution and overuse of natural resources (water) is from livestock and meat industry.

Water: 40 percent of water use in the United States is for irrigation of agricultural land and another 40 percent is for thermoelectric power. Damming the rivers for electricity deprives the land of natural water. We use "treated" water for 90 percent of our urban needs plus take in sodas, juices, sports drinks, and other sweetened liquids as a matter of habit and taste. Every snack or recreational drink neutralizes the amount of water that should be imbibed. As clean pure water is essential to the function of all cell membranes, the resulting basic dehydration is linked to poor health conditions of kidney failure, brain disease, liver dysfunction, heart disease, and accelerated ageing of the skin. We are seriously misdirecting the water supply.

Home: Soft plastics with BPA (bisphenol A) like baby bottles, food containers, water bottles now claim to be BPA free, but using BPS (bisphenol S) instead. Some flame retardants used in textiles, clothing, and household fabrics containing organo-halogens are linked to reproductive system problems. *Parabens*, a preservative found in many brands of cosmetics, body care, and some food products, *phthalates* used to make hard plastics, *dioxin* in incinerators, and released in paper and herbicide production, PCBs (polychlorinated biphenyls), heavy metals like *mercury* in fish, *arsenic* in rat bait traps, *cadmium* and *nickel* in cigarette smoke, are all endocrine-disrupting chemicals (EDC). They are similar to regular hormones and therefore able to mimic their function and block metabolic pathways. Add to the list, styrofoam containers (polystyrene), polyurethane, polyvinylchloride (PVC piping), permanent markers, and new carpets treated with formaldehyde. These everyday items are all associated with a long list of health problems: developmental delays and defects, autism, cancers, learning disabilities, impaired intelligence, low sperm counts, neurodegenerative diseases like Parkinson's and Alzheimer's, cancer, obesity, heart disease, thyroid dysfunction, allergy, asthma, insulin-resistant diabetes, and autism.

Simple activities like cooking food in aluminum foil or freezing water in reused plastic containers for drinking can lead to ingestion of toxic chemicals and long-term nervous disorders.

According to the National Cancer Institute, some 40 percent of cancers can be avoided. Pro-inflammatory foods, smoking cigarettes (toxins), excess alcohol intake (decreased immunity), drugs (legal and illegal), trauma, injury, and poor repair can all be avoided. Too much toxicity and the body cannot recover. Tolerance develops, cancer cells are triggered, become established, and the damage continues until the organ systems succumb.

Pharmaceuticals: The overuse of antibiotics in childhood and adults with viral "colds" and the use of antibiotics and hormones in livestock and poultry to ensure and enhance growth, lead to the development of drug-resistant bacteria, and rapid tolerance in human immune system. The CDC estimates that some two million people are infected by antibiotic-resistant bacteria and twenty-three thousand die each year as a direct result. Most of these deaths are in health care settings (hospitals and nursing homes).†††

The CDC released data in 2011 showing that for the first time ever in the USA, more people were killed by pharmaceutical drugs than by illegal drugs and motor vehicle accidents, and this number is increasing. The overuse of antidepressants like diethylstilbesterol (DES), mercury in antibiotic preparations, cyanide in photographic processing, strychnine in the production of medical tonics, and warfarin (a rat poison) as a blood thinner and in sugar substitutes are all detrimental to human health.

Advanced technology may be a risk factor for development of disease. High cellular phone use, social

†††   Antibiotic Resistance Threats in the United States, 2013. CDC Report.

media interaction, the LED lights from electronic devices, primarily when used at bedtime interferes with sleep rhythms by reducing melatonin levels and disrupting serotonin and neural activity and resulting in a compromised immune system.

Awareness of the presence and avoidance of these harmful products and activities is essential to disease prevention and maintenance of health and well being. Natural health strategies have a lot to offer in preventing or delaying disease formation. For example, research has shown that the main polyphenol in turmeric, called curcumin, can reverse the cancer-causing pathways that are activated by BPA in plastics. Natural products like ashwagandha, panax ginseng, astragalus, and echinacea can boost the immune system. Better quality food can provide the antioxidant protection against free radicals that are generated by many of these harmful chemicals.

Planning and practicing the six basic strategies of natural health can reduce the risks of age-related and environment generated diseases and infirmities. Most of all, positive activity will eliminate the fear of contracting and succumbing to disease.

1. Exercise/ regular physical activity

2. Basic nutrition and quality diet with adequate hydration and elimination

3. Stress management and control

4. Mental stimulation for continued brain health

5. Social connections for relaxation and peace of mind

6. Avoidance of high risk behavior and toxic environments

> Everything in excess, is opposed to nature.
>
> —Hippocrates

Vital Statistics and Lab Values as Indicators of Dysfunction

Vital statistics and laboratory values that serve as indicators of impending physiological dysfunction:

Note that the numerical values may vary between different laboratories.

It is practical to become familiar with these values.

A blood pressure reading at 120/80 is considered to be normal. Greater than 140/90 indicates hypertension. And 100/70 or below indicates hypotension.

Weight: body mass index (BMI) greater than 24 is overweight, 28 obese, 32 morbidly obese

Blood glucose: fasting blood sugar (FBS) outside the range of 70-110 or HbA1c over 6.0 indicates the status of diabetes.

Cholesterol >200 mg/dL (low density lipoprotein (LDL) >160 risky, HDL > 60 is good, + balanced ratio)

BUN (blood urea nitrogen) range 10 to 20mg percentage indicates possible liver dysfunction

Triglycerides (unsaturated vegetable oil and saturated animal fats) > 200 mg.dL

C-reactive Protein (C-RP) 10-40 mg/L (mild), 40-200 mg/L (moderate), greater than 200mg/L indicates severe infection/inflammation as in burns; or *generalized inflammation*.

Homocysteine range 10-12 mol/L indicates toxicity/ possible damage to coronary arteries

Thyroid Function tests: TSH range .5 to 5.5 (hypothyroid or hyperthyroid), also anti TG Ab, free T4, TGB

Carcinoembryonic antigen (CEA) greater than 2.5ug/L may indicate cancer

Cancer antigen (CA 125) range 40-65 U/mL is a biomarker for ovarian cancer cells

PSA 0- 4 ng/mL indicates the men's status of prostate cancer

Prothrombin time indicates status of the blood clotting system

RPR serology is a screening test for the presence or absence of venereal disease

Infections from Helicobacter pylori, herpes simplex, herpes zoster, HIV, hepatitis viruses, and toxoplasma can be identified from blood samples

Urinalysis identifies abnormalities in the urine that may indicate urinary tract infection, total body infection, kidney disease, and levels of toxins in the body

3

Natural Health Products for Disease Prevention

Natural products, fresh fruit and vegetables, whole grains, botanicals, and supplements are not a substitute for conventional medicines especially in cases of acute illness and injury. They can and should be used for prevention if the risk factors (tendency to the disease) are known and early symptoms appear, or for chronic conditions where they might be safer and in some cases, more effective over time. Once an individual is on conventional medicines for a particular condition, care should be taken not to discontinue the prescription too abruptly and follow instructions exactly as given. Some medications lose their effect, have reduced absorption, or exhibit unwanted side effects when taken with substances like milk, orange, or grapefruit juice. In many cases, both natural and conventional medicines can be used together for a determined period of time and with full awareness of the consulting and treating physicians. Be aware that many conventional medications work by stimulation or suppression, bypassing the body's own usually damaged mechanisms. Natural treatments work by attempting to restore these mechanisms and are more directed at the cause of the illness, whereas conventional medications target the symptoms of an illness, often by slowing their progress or masking their impact. If the damage is too great, the natural treatments will be unable to restore normal function on their own. Most likely, some combination of both therapy types will be needed.

Historically, pharmacologically active products can be divided into traditional, those used for thousands of years, and conventional, those in modern use. Approximately 20 percent of conventional medicines are derived from traditional sources, and 70 percent are tradition-based. When plants are manipulated and changed for health purposes, such as is done with willow bark into aspirin, cinchona into chloroquine, and the poppy into codeine, morphine, and heroin; they often become less healthy and more dangerous. As only part of the plant is used or copied, the natural balance is disrupted and invariably side effects on the receiving organism appear. In genetically engineered organisms (GMOs), the natural configuration of an organism is altered usually by the introduction of synthetic chemicals and its long-term effects are yet to be determined.

Note that natural health products in the form of "supplements" can sometimes be unreliable. Since they are not regulated by a legally sanctioned agency, the ingredients are not subject to scrutiny and may be questionable.

When using supplements, be sure to choose well-known, reputable brands.

In cases of allergy or toxic effects of conventional drugs, natural health products and traditional practices may be used alone but with full awareness that the onset and intensity of action are not the same as with the prescription medications. Research studies repeatedly confirm that the amounts required to achieve a desired effect are often too high for clinical use. However, natural products offer a more practical and safer strategy for prevention and maintenance.

Indications for the use of natural treatments include known risk factors, early symptoms, and/or intolerance of conventional treatment. For example, a newly diagnosed enlarged prostate can be reduced in size and morbidity with lycopene from cooked tomatoes and sweet red peppers, saw palmetto, pygeum, and raw garlic and prevent progression to a cancerous state. Menopausal symptoms of hot flashes and night sweats can often be allayed with vitamin E, non-GMO soy and red clover, rather than take a chance with hormone replacement therapy (HRT) in women with family histories of ovarian and uterine cancers.

Be aware that although in comparison to conventional pharmaceuticals, the side effects of botanicals are rare, but they can and do still occur. St John's wort, soy, lobelia, and chaparral have been known to have significant side effects in hypersensitive individuals or when used incorrectly.

Patients taking pharmaceutical blood thinners should be aware that natural products like ginseng, ginger, gingko biloba, and garlic have coumarin-like properties and may lead to spontaneous and excessive bleeding particularly when taken in excess or together. Ginseng and ginger can enhance small intestine transit of food when taken in small amounts, but may inhibit and block the same transit when taken in large amounts and with electrostimulation.

The effects of botanicals, whole foods, and supplements on the human body are slower in onset and less intense than those of pharmaceutical drugs. Though not meant to replace essential conventional medicines, traditional medicines and practices are often more effective in prevention of and in chronic conditions. They should be complimentary to each other.

It is recommended to take appropriate botanicals or supplements only when indicated, usually during travel when good quality whole foods may not be available, or for specific conditions where the benefits outweigh the risks. It is more important to take a supplement when there is a deficiency and the natural remedy is not available or inadequate, than to avoid taking it, such as in deficiencies of vitamin B12 and vitamin D.

Condition/Disease and Natural Products‡‡‡

The following tables include natural products that may be taken together or individually to prevent or counteract the particular disease condition. If one is prone to arthritis and gout, a combination of turmeric, boswellia, and omega-3 fish oil supplements should help allay the symptoms and reduce the underlying cause, which is inflammation. *The properties, uses, and mechanisms of actions of these natural products are all evidence-based and referenced. The dosages and amounts to be taken should be listed on the individual labels. As with all natural products and supplements, full disclosure and discussion of use should be made with your physician.*

Inflammation

Osteoarthritis, tendonitis, gout

Turmeric	Boswellia	Flaxseed	Annatto	Cayenne pepper
Cat's Claw	Spanish needle	Omega-3 fish oil	Olive oil	Apple cider vinegar

(Compare to celebrex, vioxx, ibuprofen, naproxen.)

---

‡‡‡   Associated with prevention and treatment.

Allergy

Butterbur	Anamú	Picrorhiza kurroa	Stinging nettle
Echinacea	Chamomile	Quercetin	Bromelain

(Compare to antihistamines: Claritin, Zyrtec, Allegra.)

Infection

Bacterial

Angelica	Calendula	Papaya latex	Goldenseal	Verveine
Oregano	Noni	Cloves	Garlic	Onion
Manuka honey	Guava	Wild coffee	Nutmeg	Cinnamon

(Compare to antibiotics.)

Viral

Artemesia	Lysine	Lemongrass
Gromwell	Myrrh	Olive leaf

(Compare to antivirals.)

Both Antibacterial and Antiviral

Anamú	Artemesia	Cat's claw	Cassia occidentalis	Brazil peppertree
Catuaba	Copaiba	Erva tostao	Chamomile	Garlic
Guava	Jaborandi	Mutumba	Picao preto	Ginger

Common Cold

American ginseng	Astragalus	Echinacea
Garlic	Cayenne	Zinc

(Compare to Dayquil.)

Fungal

Life plant	Melaleuca oil	Catechu	Daisy
Calendula	Poke root	Ivy	Usnea
Yawar piri piri	Manuka oil	Oregano oil	Wild yam

Parasitic

Garlic	Rue	Chaparral
Piñon colorado	Life plant	Bromelain

Immune System

Enhancers/Boosters: increase protection against infection/inflammation

Astragalus	Cat's Claw	Kelp	Onions
Echinacea	Andrographicus paniculata	Mushrooms (shiitake, reischii, maitake)	Panax ginseng
Olive leaf	Schizandra	Vitamin C	Hydraton (water)
Leeks	White teas	Cauliflower	Broccoli

Cancer

Botanicals, foods, supplements

Green tea	Anamú	Lemongrass	Graviola/soursop	Ginger	Basil
Goatweed	Turmeric	Pau d'arco	Verveine	Damiana	Chaparral
Moringa	Dandelion	Honeysuckle	Brazil nuts	Periwinkle	Cayenne
Bamboo grass	Kutaki	Noni	Turkey tail	Shiitake	Eleuthero root
Kelp/spirulina	Spanishneedle	Melatonin	Cleavers	Soy	Grapes
Flaxseed	Olive oil	Tomato	Broccoli/kale	Hops	Cereals
Legumes	Potato	Artichokes	Rosemary	Comfrey	Berries
Barberry	Pacific yew	Camptotheca	Milkweed	Maytenus	Aglaia

(Compounds from most of these natural products are in anticancer conventional drugs.)

Neurological/ Neurodegenerative

Brain and central nervous system
Dementia, Alzheimer's, Parkinsons

Coconut water	Valerian	Verveine	Lemonbalm	Vitamin E
Feverfew	Melatonin	Kava kava	Coenzyme Q10	Ashwagandha
Citocholine	Mg-L-Threonate	Eleuthero root	Omega-3 fish oil	Soy

(Compare to L-dopamine, memantine, donepezil.)

Painkillers

Cloves (*dental*)	Chanca piedra	Peekaboo plant	Pineapple (bromelain)	Guarana
Ginger	Garlic oil	Apple cider vinegar	Horseradish	Turmeric
St. John's wort	Blueberries	Mints (*all*)	Magnesium	Water (ice)

(Compare to NSAIDS like naproxen, ibuprofen.)

Anxiety

Valerian	Chamomile	Eleuthero root
Kava kava	Peppermint	Hops
Green tea (L-Threanine)	Ashwagandha	Passion flower

(Compare to diazepam, methylphenidate,
chlordiazepoxide.)

Depression

St. John's wort	S-adenosylmethionine (SAMe)	5-Hydroxytryptamine (5-HTP)

(Compare to antidepressants fluoxetine
[Prozac] and sertraline [Zoloft].)

Insomnia

Chamomile	Passionflower	Hops
Valerian	Lemonbalm	Melatonin

(Compare to zolpidem [Ambien]
and triazolam [Halcion].)

Memory

Ginkgo biloba	Ashwagandha	Thyme
Bacopa monnieri	Acetyl-L-carnitine arginate	Rosemary
Sage	DHEA	Folic acid

Stress

Panax ginseng	Eleuthero root	Schizandra	Reischii	Tulsi (holy basil)
Cordyceps	Ashwagandha	Suma	Rhodiola rosea	Chocolate

(Adaptogens/tonics compare to sertraline
and alprazolam [Xanax].)

Cardiovascular

Arjuna	Bilberry, gojiberry	Hawthornberry	Guarana
Folate	Garlic	Omega-3 fish oil	Coenzyme Q10
Lecithin	Ginkgo biloba	Coleus	Olive oil

Cholesterol

Green tea	Red wine	Red yeast rice	Ginger
Grapeseed extract	Fiber	Panax ginseng	Nuts
Grapefruit	Avocado	Oatmeal	Soy

(Compare to statins [Mevacor, Lipitor, and Zocor].)

Hypertension

Hibiscus	Anamú	Ginger
Juana la blanca	Pomegranate	Magnesium

(Compare to diuretics like chlothiazide.)

Circulation

Artinia	Ginkgo biloba	Hesperidin	Ginger
Butchers broom	Natto	Horsechestnut	Gotu kola nut
Feverfew	Mumefural	Witch hazel	Cayenne

Respiratory

COPD, Bronchitis, Emphysema

Peppermint	*Piper longum*	Slippery elm
Eucalyptus	Picrorhiza kurroa	Amor seco

Asthma

Tylophora asthmatica	Peppermint	Lobelia
Ma Huang (ephedra)	Thyme	Black tea
Inula racemosa	Omega-3 fatty acids	Turmeric

(Compare to beta agonists like albuterol and ventolin.)

Metabolic

Diabetes

Mormordica charantia	Gymnestre silvestre	Cinnamon	Vanadium
Touchi	Stevia	Vitamin B1 (thiamin)	Mulberry leaf
Red wine (resveratrol)	Chromium	Panax ginseng	Fenugreek

(Compare to metformin and humira.)

Thyroid

Bladderwrack	Seaweed products	Iodized salt	Wheatgrass

Gastrointestinal

Digestion/ Elimination

Licorice	Ginger	Turmeric	Gentian	Cayenne
Green tea	Marshmallow	Chamomile	Dandelion	Goldenseal
Anise	Plantago major	Peppermint	Probiotics	Applecider vinegar

(Compare to antacids like Zantac and Prilosec.)
Emesis (Vomiting)

Cloves	Peppermint	Ipecac
Peach	Raspberry leaf tea	Ginger
Apple cider vinegar	Water (electrolytes)	Fennel tea

Constipation

Aloe vera juice	Turkey rhubarb	Olive oil
Fiber	Cascara sagrada	Psyllium
Flaxseed	Prunes	Gentian

Diarrhea

Guava	Peach leaf extract	Pigeon peas leaf tea
Banana	Sweet potato	Pumpkin mash

Liver

Milk thistle	Yellow dock	Picrorhiza kurroa	Dandelion
Parsley	Kelp	Wasabi	Plantago major
Hydrangea	Artichoke	Reischii mushroom	Shiitake mushroom
Kutaki	Trimethylglycine	Kinski	Goldenseal
Calcium-D-glucarate	Garlic	Grapefruit	Beets/carrots

Blood Purifiers

Burdock	Dandelion	Rue
Goldenseal	Sarsaparilla	Chaparral

Genitourinary

Cranberry	Cayenne pepper	Fenugreek
Celery seed	Green tea	Stinging nettle root
Blueberry	Bromelain/ choline enzymes	Garlic

Kidney Stones (Urolithiasis)

Cane piece senna	Uva ursi	Dandelion root
Pomegranate	Magnesium	Lemon, olive oil, AC vinegar

Bladder and Kidney Infection (Cystitis, Pyelonephritis)

Uva ursi	Dandelion root	Cranberry	Water (hydration)

Yeast Infection (*Candida albicans*)

Lactobacillus probiotic	Tea tree oil	Boric acid	Jatoba

Musculoskeletal

Bone and Cartilage Health

S-adenosylmethionine (SAMe)	Willow bark	Glucosamine/chondroitin
Red clover	Methylsulfonylmethane (MSM)	Olive oil

Women's Health

PMS/ Dysmenorrhea: Evening primrose oil
Pregnancy: Abuta Shatavari
Post-partum: Angelica root
Menopause

Black cohosh	Magnesium/ calcium	Red clover	Blue cohosh
Wild yam	Vitamin E	Vitex	Hops
Soy	Dong quai	Ginger	Maca root

Men's Health

Benign Prostatic Hypertrophy

Saw palmetto	Panax ginseng	Jatoba
Selenium	Pumpkin seed oil	Lycopene
Pink grapefruit	Watermelon	Guava
Pomegranate	Betasitosterol	Zinc

Impotence/Erectile Dysfunction

Oysters	Celery	Almonds
Avocado	Figs	Garlic
Chocolate	Maca root	Yohimbe

Eye Health
(antioxidants for cataracts, macular degeneration, glaucoma)

Bilberry	Jaborandi	Chrysanthemum	Cannabis sativa
Grapeseed extract	Carnitine	Lutein	Zeaxanthin
Vitamin C	Sulfur compounds	Flaxseed	Zinc

Skin/Dermal

Aloe vera gel	Arnica	Calendula
Tea tree oil	St. Johns wort	Sangre de grado
Chamomile	Lemonbalm	Lavender
Manuka oil	Castor oil	Coconut oil

Mucosal / Dental
Pharyngitis (sore throat) / Gingivitis (gum disease)

licorice gargle	Honey	Calendula oil	Salt water gargle
Marshmallow root	Cayenne	Slippery elm	Myrrh
Coconut oil (raw)	Sesame seed oil	Sage and Echinacea	Peppermint

Ears
Otitis media, tinnitus, hearing loss

Mullein and garlic oil	Elderberry syrup	Ginkgo biloba	Vit. A (cod liver oil)	vinpocetine

Nose

(Compare to painkillers, decongestants,
antibiotics, steroids.)
Epistaxis, chronic sinusitis, chronic rhinitis (see allergy)

Mushrooms	Capsaicin spray	Salt water irrigation
Peppermint	Eucalyptus	Humidity (humidifier)
Horseradish	Yarrow	Warm water heat application

Weight Loss

Garcinia cambrogia	Borage oil	Dandelion	Hoodia gorgoni
Brewers yeast	Kola nut	Green coffee bean	Panax ginseng

Basic Nutritional Food Groups

Fats are mainly linolenic and linoleic acids and triglycerides. Plant-based fats, like olive oil, that are liquid at room temperature are unsaturated. Animal-based fats, like fat rind on a steak, that are solid at room temperature are saturated. Unsaturated fats are healthier than saturated fats. Omega-3 fatty acids that regulate cholesterol metabolism are a precursor of prostaglandins and the main storage form of energy in the body. They are polyunsaturated.

Good Fats

Avocado	Flaxseed	Cold water fish	Extra-virgin olive oil	Nuts
Cheese	Yogurt	Coconut oil	Dark chocolate	Whole eggs

Carbohydrates provide the body with the energy from glucose it needs to function properly.

Fiber	Whole grain	Cereals
Brown sugar	Seeds/nuts	Fruit
Vegetables	Honey	Legumes

Proteins consist of nitrogen-based amino acids, which provide the structural components of most body tissues, as well as enzymes, blood cells, and antibodies.

Soy (non-GMO)	Legumes/ lentils	Beans	Fish
Poultry	Bromelain/ papain	Whole eggs	Lean pork

Antioxidants

Free radicals are potentially dangerous molecules that are formed in the body from chemical reactions that leave them in need of an ionizing electron. When allowed to interact with normal cells, free radical molecules take the electron they need from the normal cell, thereby damaging DNA and causing cell death (apoptosis). *Antioxidants* are natural products that neutralize or block the harmful activity of free radical molecules by donating an electron to the unstable structure. Foods with high levels of antioxidant activity include vitamins A,C, and E; vegetables like spinach, artichokes, okra, kale, potatoes, and broccoli; fruit like berries, pears, apples, grapes; whole grains like oats, wheat, rye, barley, buckwheat, quinoa; nuts like walnuts, pecans, hazelnuts, almonds, with selenium; and dark chocolate, red wine, coffee, and herbal teas.

Twelve Superfoods with High Levels of Beneficial Antioxidants

Broccoli	Salmon	Eggs	Yogurt
Beans	Walnuts	Oatmeal	Olive oil
Blueberries	Quinoa	Dark chocolate (>70%)	Herbal teas

Eating real whole fresh food is the best, nutritional health-promoting strategy on the planet.

Natural Products for Good Health

Natural products contain multiple chemicals made by plants or occurring in nature to benefit the health of the organism. Only a relatively small sampling of natural products appears here to correlate with the previous listing and to compliment the next chapter, which presents specific strategies for prevention and natural treatment of disease. The ones starred (*) are suggested for good health maintenance and should be used on a regular or daily basis. These products are listed with the chief chemical ingredients correlated with its main use and effect, suggested dosage where available, and adverse effects if present. They are accompanied with reference numbers when verification is desired.

Alpha lipoic acid is an essential fatty acid, part of the omega 3 group with strong antioxidant activity which sustains and improves nerve cell (neuron) function. It reduces the pain of diabetic peripheral neuropathy and other neurological diseases. The average dosage is 600 to 1200mg daily, and it can be found in natural broccoli, spinach, potatoes, liver and kidney organs, and yeast.[1]

Aloe vera has seventy-six glycosides, fifteen alkaloids, and four plant steroids. The skin moisturizers, acemannan polysaccharide, aloe-emodin, auxins, and gibberellins in the inner gel, contribute to wound healing and inflammation control. It has anthraquinones, salicylic acid, and saponins which act as antibiotics, antivirals, antiseptics, and analgesics. Liberal topical application is used for inflammation or infection, like skin rash, gingivitis, psoriasis, lichen planus, eczema, burns, and genital herpes. It has minerals, vitamins, and enzymes in the liquid which act as purgatives and laxatives. The recommended dosage is a mixture of two teaspoons of fresh aloe vera gel, with or without honey and thirty to forty milliliter of fruit juice in a blender. Varying dosages can be used for constipation, heart disease, high cholesterol, inflammatory bowel syndrome (ulcerative colitis), diabetes, and liver disease. Aloe treatments can be used two to three times daily for two to twenty weeks or until the condition is healed.[2, 3]

Anamú (*Petiveria allicea*) has astilbin, benzaldehyde, dibenzyl trisulfide, and many antioxidants, which kill cancer cells and block inflammation at the first stages, especially in arthritis. It is used as a painkiller, an antibiotic, antiviral against colds and flu with fever, antifungal, immune system enhancer, and diuretic. It should not be used in pregnancy as it may induce abortion. It also has blood sugar lowering and thinning effects so should be taken with caution in individuals with diabetes and/or using coumarin. The dried whole plant is taken as a tea, one cup two to three times daily.[4]

Anise (*Pimpinella anisum*) is a licorice-based plant with anethole, estragole, and many antioxidants. It is used as a flavoring, digestive aid, antifungal, diuretic, and aperitif in liquors. The seeds may be used in a cup of tea to settle an upset stomach as needed.[5]

*****Apple cider vinegar** from organically grown apples contains acetic acid (from fermented sugar, alcohol, and yeast), which is antibacterial, antiseptic, and anti-inflammatory, helps to lower blood sugar, contributes to weight loss, and is a good detoxification for gout. It also contains malic acid and pectin, which are good for blood pressure and cholesterol control. With a high level of ash, which alkalinizes the body, it is active against cancer cells that thrive in an acid environment. A regular dose contributes to prevention of inflammations like rhinitis, gingivitis, pharyngitis, and gout. The average dosage is one teaspoon three times daily.[6]

AREDS eye formula is a combination of vitamins and minerals that are connected with eye health: zinc, 80mg (helps create protective melanin pigment); vitamin C, 500mg (antioxidant protection from UV damage, promotes capillary blood vessel health, helps with iron absorption); vitamin E, 400 IU (reduces progression of macular degeneration and cataract formation); copper, 2mg (antioxidant inhibition of progression of macular degeneration); lutein, 10mg; and zeaxanthin, 2mg (are macular pigments that protect the retina and macula from harmful UV radiation). These antioxidants can be found in most fresh fruit and vegetables and should be taken as four to five servings daily. Supplement dosage with capsules is one to two a day.[7]

Arginine (amino acid**)** to make proteins, high-caloric foods like eggs, meats, dairy, and fat-rich foods like peanuts, seeds, coconut oil, gelatin, oats, and whole wheat. It is a precursor to nitrous oxide, which relaxes and expands narrow blood vessels and increases blood flow. Used for treating congestive heart failure, angina, erectile dysfunction, and prevention of Alzheimer's by blocking the formation of plaques and tangles, considered to be "brain protective." Caution: as too much intake may exacerbate Herpes simplex conditions.[8]

Arnica (*A. montana*) is a mountain flowering plant that contains sesquiterpene lactones, thymol, and helenalin, which release compounds to reduce swelling, improve circulation in damaged tissue, boost flow of nutrients, and flush out damaged blood from the wound. It is applied on bruises, hematomas, ecchymoses, after blunt trauma, muscle soreness, sprain, and spasm, and abscess. Used only on closed wounds, it is toxic when taken internally. Homeopathic dosages are available.[9]

Artemesia (*A. annua*) is a wormwood plant originally from China, with artemesinin, sesquiterpene lactones and tannins, which kill parasites when inside red blood cells as in malaria, is antiviral against bird flu, and has a strong antioxidant activity against cancer and general inflammatory diseases. Tea infusions and dried leaves have shown preventive and effective treatment results. It may also be taken in capsule form in combination with other antimicrobials.[10]

Artichoke (*Cynara cardunculus*) contains polyphenols (cynarine, apigenin, and luteolin) with high antioxidant activity, plus vitamins, minerals, fats, carbohydrates; digestive aid (dyspepsia, IBS) , liver, and gallbladder function, raises HDL and LDL ratio that reduces cholesterol levels (by inhibiting HMG-CoA reductase), which reduces the risk of arteriosclerosis and coronary heart disease.[11]

Artinia (N-Acetyl D-Glucosamine Chitin-Glucan) is a vegetable fiber-derived nutraceutical from the fungus *Aspergillus niger bacillus* that promotes natural antioxidant defenses that help maintain cholesterol levels and promote arterial cardiovascular health. The dose is 750mg, twice daily.[12]

Ashwagandha (*Withania somnifera*) has been used for thousands of years in ayurveda to treat neurological disorders characterized by effects of oxidative stress on the brain. Its main constituent, withanolides, has been shown to offset fatigue, memory loss, and motor effects of Parkinson's disease. It is often taken as a nerve tonic and memory enhancer. The dose is 500mg twice daily.[13]

Astragalus (*A. membrannacaeus*) is a traditional Chinese medicine with high levels of polysaccharides acting as antioxidants that stimulate the immune system, inhibit chemically-induced immunosuppression and kills cancer cells. Helping to protect the body against physical, mental, and emotional stress, it is used as an adaptogen tonic against liver disease, debilitating colds and flu, the effects of diabetes and hypertension and cancer. The dose is 250 to 500mg three to four times a day, depending on level of the condition (1000mg). In fu-zheng therapy for established cancer the dose is higher at 1000 to 1500mg a day, or tincture (1:5) 3ml , two to three times a day for stimulation of white blood cells during chemotherapy.[14]

*Avocado (*Persea americana*) contains catechins, oleic acids, monounsaturated fats, and lots of fiber, which work to lower LDL cholesterol and raise HDL (good) cholesterol. It acts against the inflammation of arthritis, psoriasis, and eczema as well as hypertension through its diuretic action. When in season eating an avocado daily is a healthy addition to many meals.[15a, b]

Bacopa monnieri offers protection from neurodegeneration, reduction of anxiety, and restoration of cognitive function through its bacopaside and alkaloids constituents, which increase blood flow within the brain. Excessive doses may lead to elevated thyroxine and upset gastrointestinal system from increased peristalsis. The standard supplement dosage is 300mg daily.[16a]

Bamboo grass of the Poaceae family, contains phytosterols like chlorophyll, which has antimutagenic activity, plus fiber, flavones,vitamins, and minerals. Taken as a drink along with other chlorophylls, it is an effective preventative against cancers of the breast and colon and immunity booster.[16b]

Basil (*Ocimum basilicum*) contains eugenol, citrals, linalool, apigenin, and other essential oils that give it strong antioxidant as well as antibacterial, anticancer, and antiviral properties. Holy basil (*O.sanctum*) is a variant with antistress properties by modulation of brain monoamines. Both are effective against herpes and adenoviral infections. In Puerto Rico, the plant has been used after delivery to increase lactation. Fresh or dried leaves may be used in cooking for preventive measures. The standard dosage is 1 to 2 grams of leaves. Due to potential toxicity of the oils, basil should not be used during pregnancy.[17a, b]

*Berries are generally very strong antioxidants containing polyphenols, anthrocyanins, and flavonoids. All berries are beneficial for disease prevention. Blueberries, blackberries, cranberries, raspberries, strawberries, bayberries, and goji berries all have phytochemicals that are anticancer, antibacterial, and antiviral.

Bilberry (*Vaccinium myrtillus*) has a special affinity for the eyes. With its high antioxidant content of anthocyanadins and polyphenols, it protects the retinal photoreceptors against UV light damage, protects the lens of the eye against rapid cataract formation and stabilizes retinal small blood vessel membranes. Standard dosage is 25mg per day orally or a handful with cereal or in a fresh fruit bowl. [18a, b]

Black cohosh (*Cimicifuga racemosa*, synonym, *Actea racemosa*) has phytochemicals that mimic the effects of estrogen, without the unwanted side effects. It can treat or prevent some of the symptoms of menopause, like hot flashes, excessive sweating, palpitations, vaginal dryness, and mood disturbances. It should not be given to children, or during pregnancy and lactation due to its effects on sex hormones. The recommended dose is between 40 to 80mg per day.[19]

Black tea (*Camillia sinensis*) is green tea whose leaves have been oxidized. It contains caffeine, theophylline, and catechins, which provide central nervous system stimulation and asthma control. With powerful antioxidants, it offers some protection against ovarian cancer, diabetes, cholesterol, and kidney stones. A good dosage is two cups a day plain. Agave syrup, honey of stevia may be used but no sugar.[20]

Blueberry (*Vaccinium corymbosum*) is high in antioxidants, particularly anthocyanins, which is second only to cranberry in protecting the bladder and urinary tract from infections. It is very protective of the retinas of the eyes from UV radiation. Its epicatechins enhance growth of blood vessels and nerve cells to maturity, which is very preventive of age related degenerations.[21]

Boswellia (*Boswellia serrata*), also known as Indian frankincense, contains boswellic acid and many triterpenic acids, which block the classic inflammation pathway, thereby reducing the inflammation and pain of osteoarthritis. It is also effective against ulcerative colitis and Crohn's disease. It works like NSAIDS, but without the side effects. The standard dosage is 400 to 1,200mg a day orally or may be used as a topical gel.[22]

*Broccoli (*Brassica oleracea*) contains essential nutrients and therapeutic phytochemicals, sulforaphane, isothiocyanates, and indole-3-carbinols, which inhibits cell proliferations of several cancers, inflammatory diseases (osteoarthritis, Crohn's), and heart disease. With high levels of vitamin C, vitamin A, zinc, and fiber, it is a true chemoprevention antioxidant. A cruciferous vegetable should be taken in on a daily basis.[23]

Butchers broom (*Rusci aculeatus*) is a relative of asparagus and contains saponins and esculin, which constrict blood vessels especially in the lower extremities. It improves the circulation and prevent clots from the pooling of blood. It is useful for preventing and treating hemorrhoids, varicose veins, and atherosclerosis (hardening of the arteries of the heart). The shoots may be eaten raw or the roots cooked much like asparagus. It is available in capsule form or topical cream.[24]

Butterbur (*Petasites hybridus*) is effective against the symptoms of allergic rhinitis and reduces the frequency and severity of migraine attacks, by its action on the inflammatory response of white blood cells. It does not have the side effects of the conventional antihistamines. A standard dosage is 50 to 75 mg twice daily when in season for prevention and four times daily when affected.[25]

*Calcium is a mineral nutrient required for many cellular processes, bone and teeth health early and late in life. Deficiencies may lead to osteoporosis, poor blood clotting, accelerated tooth decay, rickets, and increased risk of bone fractures. The standard dosage for men with deficiency is 1,200 mg daily and for women and the elderly, 1,800mg a day. Cold water fish like salmon, dairy products like milk and cheese, vegetables like broccoli, kelp, and kale, beans, nuts, and fortified cereals are good sources. Vitamin D is needed to absorb calcium.[26]

Calendula *(C. officinalis)* or marigold flower contains a large number of antioxidant phytochemicals, which promote their activity against skin infections with bacteria and fungi. It has excellent wound healing properties for burns, abrasions, and rashes. Topically, it is used as an oil, cream, or lotion. It can be ingested internally in diluted form for liver and kidney antioxidant protection.[27]

Cannabis sativa with its high levels of THC and other cannabinoid plants with more CBD are increasingly being used for medical purposes. In measured doses and perhaps in a soon to be available spray form, marijuana can be used for epilepsy, digestive disorders, to relieve effects of chemotherapy for cancer, and for relief of symptoms of neurodegenerative disorders, like Parkinson's and multiple sclerosis.[28]

Cat's Claw (*Uncaria tomentosa*) is a special "teaching" plant of the Amazon, with a combination of oxidole alkaloids, carboxyalkylesters, glycosides, tannins, and catechins, which are strongly anti-inflammatory, antibacterial, antiviral, and anticancer that block the inflammation pathway at several crucial points that prevent heat, redness, pain, and swelling. It is a climbing vine whose stem contains the highest levels of active phytochemicals. The standard dosage is 250 to 1,000mg a day.[29]

Cayenne (*Capsicum annum frutescens*) or chili pepper contains capsaicin, which reduces pain by depleting nerve endings of the chemical (substance P) that causes it. Along with other capsaicinoids with antioxidant activity, it is used as an analgesic to relieve the pain of arthritis, for protection and healing of gastric ulcers, to lower the risk of prostate cancer by reducing inflammation, to prevent kidney and gall stones, and protect the heart. The standard dosage is forty thousand units or 30 to 250mg daily, depending on the condition and stage. It is an excellent spice for cooking many dishes.[30]

Celery seed (*Apium graveolens*) has antimicrobial , parasiticidal antiviral, and repellant properties. Along with several other seeds and spice plants (fennel, basil, oregano, cumin, rosemary), it inhibits the P450 cytochrome system in the intestines to promote good gut bacteria and permit absorption of nutrients.[31]

Cereal grains, whole grains, pasta, and brown rice intake is directly associated with reduced risk of death by diabetes and cancer (but not heart and respiratory disease and infections). High in fiber, protein, antioxidants, B vitamins, the intake of three servings a day is associated with reduced cholesterol levels and obesity, regular bowel movements, and good gastrointestinal health.[32]

Chamomile (*Matricaria recrutita*) contains essential oils with properties that aid digestion, lower cholesterol, promote skin healing, treat parasites (acarids and mites), viral infections with herpes simplex, and is antibacterial, antiallergenic and anticancer. It is especially effective as a tonic for children's colic at a dosage of 150ml per cup three times a day. At a dose of 200mg/kg in animal studies, it has demonstrated anticonvulsive properties by increasing the time between seizure attacks.[33a, b]

Chocolate (*Theobroma cacao*) contains energy-rich polyphenols, which reduce stress, especially in females and at the same time, may act as a mild stimulant due to its theobromine and caffeine content. Its anthocyanins act as antioxidants to reduce free radicals and allow nitric oxide, a blood vessel-dilating chemical, to achieve higher levels, which may help with ED problems. Its flavanols and procyanins inhibit the growth of human colon cancer cells and demonstrate anti inflammation activity. The effective dose is 40 grams of dark chocolate daily. Caution: commercial chocolate with high levels of cocoa butter, fat, sugars, and milk increases the risk of obesity and tooth decay.[34a, b, c]

Chromium supplementation for type 2 diabetes remains controversial. Some studies show that 200 mcg twice a day is beneficial in elderly diabetics, while other studies appear to be are inconclusive.[35]

Cinchona bark from which the alkaloid, quinine, is derived is still the prototype of antimalarial medicines. It also contains quinidine for heart arrhythmias. Chloroquine prophylaxis dosage for malaria is 300 mg once a week prior to travel to an endemic area, and once a week during and for four weeks after.[36]

Cinnamon (*Cinnamomum verum*) contains cinnamic acid, cinnulin, eugenol, and several diterpenes that have antibacterial, antifungal, antioxidant, detoxification, digestive, blood thinning, and blood sugar lowering activities. Effective dosage has not been established but 1 to 2 grams of powder a day is considered to be safe. High doses may be toxic.[37]

Cloves (*Eugenia aromatic*) and clove oil with eugenol, eugenyl acetate, and methyl salicylate, is effective in the treatment of dental pain, cough suppression, and indigestion. Chewing a few cloves imparts analgesia to the mouth and teeth. A few cloves in tea may settle the stomach and may quiet a dry cough.[38]

Coca (*Erythroxylum coca or novogranatense*) is particularly effective against altitude sickness due to its blood vessel constriction activity. It may also be used as an anesthetic, analgesic, for relief of headache pain, gastrointestinal upset, and motion sickness. Chewing the leaf, tea, chewing gum, and candy are several ways of ingesting coca. When taken in leaf form, there is no toxicity nor addiction.[39a, b]

*****Coconut** (*Cocos nucifera*) is a fruit (drupe) not a nut and is valued for its water, milk, oil, and butter, which contain good fats. High in the amino acid, arginine, it can block the damage to brain cells in early Alzheimers's disease and actually improve cognitive function. Its array of essential fatty acids includes gamma linolenic acid (GLA) and eicosapentanoic acid (EPA) that inhibit invasion and metastasis of some cancer cells. It is effective in rewetting dry eyes. Though loaded with saturated fats itself, two tablespoons a day (30ml) is purported to help lose belly fat. Topical application helps promote wound healing (burns) by increasing re-epithelialization, improving antioxidant activity, and stimulating collagen repair mechanisms. The therapeutic dosage is one tablespoon for cooking, added to food or in cereal, and one drop to each eye as needed.[40a, b]

Coenzyme Q10 (*ubiquinone*) is a natural antioxidant substance in cellular mitochondria, which contributes to energy production within cells, resulting in boosting circulation and regulating the immune system. It is beneficial for heart health by improving levels of lipids (HDL and HDL/LDL ratios) that contribute to prevention of angina, congestive heart failure, arrhythmias, and high blood pressure. It influences gingivitis, migraine attacks, breast cancer recurrence prevention, and maintains normal pregnancy. Organs with Coenzyme Q10 are kidney, heart, and liver, which require high energy levels. Foods with coenzyme q10 are broccoli, sulfurous, dark, leafy greens like broccoli, nuts, fish, pork, chicken, beef...but not enough to sustain adequate blood levels... The recommended additional dosage is 90 to 200mg daily.[41]

Coffee (*Caffea arabica*) contains caffeine, theobromine, and antioxidants, which stimulate brain cells to make serotonin and dopamine, effective antidepressants. In addition to preventing type 2 diabetes, lowering the risk of liver disease, reliving migraine attacks, alleviating the movements of Parkinson's, it is reported to protect against heart attack. Caution: more than two cups a day can cause anxiety, severe irritability, increased blood pressure and heart rate, severe dehydration, osteoporosis through loss of calcium, fluctuations in blood sugar, weight gain associated with increased need for sugary snacks and dependence/addiction.[42]

Coleus (*C. forskohlii*) contains forskohlin in its roots, which relaxes heart muscles, dilates, and widens blood vessels leading to decreased blood pressure and relief of heart failure and angina. By increasing levels of cyclic AMP it relaxes muscles of the bronchioles in the lungs to offer relief of asthma and enable easier breathing. It has been used in IV form for idiopathic congestive cardiopathy (heart disease) and inhaled in powder form for asthma.[43]

Comfrey *(Symphytum off.)* contains allantoin and pyrrolizine alkaloids, which reduce inflammation and stimulate repair and healing of damaged tissues, like bones and skin. It is also effective with back pain, osteoarthritis, and large abrasions. Use topically. Internal use can lead to liver damage.[44]

***Cordyceps** (C. sinensis)* is a Chinese mushroom grown on caterpillars, which shows strong antimicrobial activity against a broad spectrum of bacteria and fungi, and cytotoxic properties against several tumors. It boosts the immune system and has antioxidant activity against scavenging radicals, reducing power and chelating ability on iron ions. It can be used to reduce fatigue and boost energy by enhancing lung function. It can treat cancer. It is available in capsules, tinctures, solutions, powder and dried (tea), 5 to 10 grams a day. Caution: when using blood thinners and it may increase testosterone levels.[45]

Cranberry (*Vaccinium macrocarpon* and *oxycoccus*) is loaded with anthocyanidins, flavonoids, vitamin C and E, fiber, and manganese. With very high antioxidant levels, it prevents uric acid and bacteria from adhering to bladder walls, prevents the formation of stones and reduces risk of proteus bacterial infection. It is a very effective deterrent to kidney and bladder infections and cancers. Drinking eight to sixteen ounces three to four times a week, plus eating fresh or dried cranberries is good.[46]

Damiana (*Turnera diffusa*) contains arbutin, alkaloids, terpenes, and volatile oils, which affect the central nervous system directly to reduce anxiety, raise testosterone and estrogen levels, reduce inflammation in the reproductive organs, and boost energy. The leaves dried and steeped into a tea.[47]

Dandelion (*Taxacum officinalis*) contains more carotenoids than carrots, B, C, and E vitamins, luteolin, and calcium for bone health. By its antioxidant effect of reducing and blocking oxidative stress in cells, it detoxifies and purges the liver, gall bladder, and bowels. It has scavenger activity in blocking cancer cells, removing excess sugar from the blood, lowers blood pressure by diuresis, and its high fiber composition reduces the frequency of constipation. It may be taken as fresh leaves in salad or as capsules.[48]

DHEA (*Dehydroepiandrosterone*) a precursor for testosterone and estradiol, an adrenal hormone, naturally decreases with age. It can be used to prevent memory loss, assist erectile dysfunction, and to treat lupus erythematosus. Supplemental DHEA increases testosterone levels in middle-aged men, which may increase the risk of prostate cancer.[49a, b]

Dong quai (*Angelica sinensis*) has been a vital part of traditional Chinese medicine for two thousand years. Related to carrots, parsley, dill, and celery, it has protective effects against oxidative stress and displays anti inflammation and antispasmodic properties. It is best used for menstrual irregularities, pelvic pain, and fatigue. Caution: Being estrogenic, it may lead to uterine contractions so should be avoided in pregnancy. The standard dose is 2,000 to 4,000 mg a day when and as needed.[50]

Echinacea (*E. purpura*) is indicated for acute viral infections like colds and flu. It contains phenols, polysaccharides, acids, and alkaloids, which regulate the inflammatory response to viruses and bacteria, by increasing the number of T cells. As a blood purifier, it expels toxins and poisons and has an anticancer property of inhibiting tumor cells. When combined with goldenseal, it is especially effective against influenza flu and common colds in the acute phase by regulating T cell number and function. It is most effective in acute situations at a dosage of 6 to 9 grams per day for up to three days.[51]

Eggs are a low-calorie food with high nutritional value. Loaded with protein, fat, vitamins (especially riboflavin), and minerals (especially iron, phosphorus, and the antioxidant, selenium), eggs are high in cholesterol but don't raise cholesterol levels in the blood. The liver reduces its production of cholesterol when eggs are eaten. Caution: some 30 percent of people are responders with gene type (ApoE4) that will allow for cholesterol increase when eggs and other fats are eaten. Eggs raise the HDL cholesterol, which reduces the risk of heart disease; contain choline, which builds cell membranes and produces signaling molecules in the brain; change small LDL cholesterol to large LDL cholesterol, which is less dangerous to blood vessels; contain lutein and zeaxanthin in the yolk, which are strong antioxidants specific for eye health (retina) and decreased rick of cataract formation; and have quality protein with amino acids which are essential for building cells and metabolic functions.[52]

Elderberry (*Sambucus nigra*) can be taken as a juice, syrup, tea, jelly, liquor, or wine mostly made from the flowers. It contains cyanogenic glycosides in all the green parts so is very poisonous. The berries should be cooked. It inhibits the influenza virus A and B to reduce the cough symptoms and clear the ears and throat much better than placebo. As an immune system booster, it is effective against both viruses and bacteria in reducing inflammation.[53]

Eleuthero root (*Eleutherococcus senticossus*), or Siberian ginseng, is an adaptogen, which contains eleutherosides A and B, strong antioxidants that relax the endothelial cell walls of blood vessels and inhibit potassium channels to produce an antianxiety, antidepressant effect. S an immune system booster, it helps to offset the bone marrow damage from chemotherapy. It is used as a natural treatment for stress, especially strenuous aerobic activity. The standard dosage is 300 to 1,200 mg a day.[54]

Ephedra (*E. sinica*) also known as Ma huang, is an adrenalin analog much like amphetamine, which is used for weight loss, asthma attacks, bronchitis, relief of lung congestion, cough suppressant, and energy booster. In high doses and hypersensitive individuals it can be very toxic. Caution: The adverse effects include irritability, anxiety, hyperactivity, intense sweating, insomnia, and death. Over-the-counter availability is currently banned in the USA. Standard dosage is less than 30 mg per day.[55]

Eucalyptus *(E. globulus)* is a genus of trees with over seven hundred species, most of which are native to Australia. Containing terpenoids and volatile oils, it has many economic uses, from construction to biofuels and insect repellants. With antibiotic and antioxidant activities, the oil can be used in food supplements, cough syrups, toothpaste, antiseptics, and decongestants. Dosages are small and based on needs.[56]

Evening primrose oil (*Oenothera biennis*) from the seeds contains fatty acids that decrease inflammation and can be used as a moisturizer. Research shows that it appears to work best in combination with other omega-3 fatty acids to reduce diabetic nerve pain, arthritis pain, and slow the progression of osteoporosis. The standard dose is from 500mg to 3grams daily.[57]

Fennel (*Foeniculum vulgare*) is high in antioxidants (flavonoids, phenolics) fatty acids, proteins, and coumarins, which give it antibiotic and liver protection properties. Primarily a culinary spice, it can be used to treat fever, digestive problems, prevent blood clots, and kill cancer cells.[58]

Fenugreek (*Trigonella foenumgraecum*) is an Asian plant whose leaves and seeds are used in culinary dishes. The chemical, Sotolon, gives it a sweet smell. By raising free testosterone levels in the blood, it is used for erectile dysfunction and increasing sexual desires in men and women. By slowing the absorption of sugar in the stomach and stimulating the release of insulin, it has been used for lowering blood sugar in type 2 diabetics. Dosage depends on the vital statistics of the user, health, age, purpose, etc.[59]

Feverfew (*Tanacetum parthenium*) contains flavonoid glycosides, terpenoids, and pinenes, which decrease inflammation in joints (arthritis) by blocking the release of white blood cells in response to challenge and regulating blood vessel tone. It has strong antioxidant activity in preventing and treating migraine headaches. The dosage varies depending on the manufacturer, 50 to 150mg of dried leaves. Caution as too high a dose or sensitivity may cause allergic reactions of skin as well as gastrointestinal upset. It may interact with blood thinners to cause bleeding.[60]

***Fiber**, both soluble and insoluble, in the diet influences and promotes digestion, laxation, prevents disease by regulating gut bacteria and microflora, regulates pancreatic and liver functions, promotes weight loss and cardiovascular health, and lowers risk of type 2 diabetes, colon and breast cancers. Included are whole grains, beans, nuts, fruit like apples and plums, potatoes, dark leafy greens, yellow vegetables like zucchini and squash, plus plants like psyllium, hyssop, alfalfa, rhubarb, and many more. The normal intake for preventive medicine should be around 20 to 30 grams or four servings daily. For established cancer, hepatitis, diabetes, irritable bowel disease and heart disease, increase the intake to 40 grams daily and must be accompanied by adequate water intake.[61]

***Flaxseed** oil or seed is a functional antioxidant food and a main source of omega-3 fatty acids and lignans. Also containing phenolic glycosides, vitamins, and minerals, it lowers LDL cholesterol, reduces risk of breast and prostate cancers, reduces severity of diabetes, decreases the concentration of pro-inflammatory proteins, reduces high blood pressure by action on the peripheral blood vessels, and promotes bowel movements. It may be taken internally as tea, oils, seed, and externally in cream, oil or ointment form. Caution: without adequate water intake, too much flaxseed may result in bowel obstruction.[62]

***Folate** (folic acid), vitamin B9, is involved in the synthesis of major amino acids, adenosine, guanine, and thymidine required for making DNA. Adequate intake can reduce homocysteine levels, which contribute to heart health, growth, and reproduction, early embryonic development especially neurological, reduction of anxiety, depression, gout, and prevention of atherosclerosis and colon cancer. Foods high in folic acid include broccoli, asparagus, citrus fruit, legumes, avocado, and okra. Folate supplements are recommended in pregnancy and deficiency anemias. A daily dosage of 1 milligram is required for normal function. Steaming of food (vegetables) can keep more folate content.[63]

Foxglove *(Digitalis purpura)* includes some twenty different species of plants, all with some forms of digitalin, the active ingredient from which many heart medicines are derived. The cardiac glycosides from these medicines are used to regulate heart rhythm and treat congestive heart failure through regulation of calcium contents in contractile heart muscles. Caution: an overdose of digitalis can cause nausea, vomiting, diarrhea and yellow vision (xanthopsia). Dosages should be set and regulated by a physician.[64]

Garcinia cambrogia is the fruit of the *garcinia gummagutta* tree, also known as Malabar tamarind, which is marketed primarily for weight loss. The active ingredient in the fruit rind, hydroxycitric acid, blocks the production of fat, increase fat oxidation and increases brain serotonin levels, which reduce the feelings of hunger. It also has many xanthones, benzophenones, and organic acids which serve to reduce LDL cholesterol and increase HDL. A safe dosage is 500 to 1500 mg daily, and it will probably take a "good while" to lose the weight.[65]

*Garlic (*Allium sativa*) contains allin and allinase which when chopped or minced converts to allicin, the active ingredient, which is a powerful antibacterial, antiviral, antifungal, immune boosting anticancer natural through its antioxidant/anti-inflammation activities. When chopped or minced or crushed it becomes diallyl disulfide and other organosulfur compounds, which are garlic's own defense against pests. It reduces arteriosclerosis and fat deposition in the arteries, normalizes lipoproteins and blood pressure, and prevents thrombosis. Studies show that allicin may be effective in the treatment of resistant bacteria (MRSA). One clove a day is very wise preventive medicine.[66a, b]

Gentian (*Gentiana lutea or crinita*) contains specialized gentopicrosides, amarogentin, and xanthones which kill bacteria and parasitic worms directly. It is used to prevent and treat gaseous indigestion (dyspepsia) gastritis and for appetite stimulation. It enhances liver and gall bladder function and treats fevers and colds, especially associated with the digestive system. Dosage may be by digestive tonic of 1 to 4 grams per day. Caution: it should not be used in cases of gastrointestinal ulcers or hypertension.[67]

*Ginger (*Zinziber officinalis*) is one of the wonder roots of the world. It can be taken as capsules, tea, ginger ale, candied ginger or powder in doses usually of one to two teaspoons daily or one capsule up to four times a day, as needed. As an excellent spice in cooking stews, its array of acids, phenolic antioxidants, gingerols, shagaols, and terpenoids have strong effects on the inflammation pathway, pain signaling, and enzyme activity. It reduces the nausea of chemotherapy, motion and morning sickness, heals and protects the gut mucosa, promotes probiotics growth, assists with peristalsis in digestion, lowers cholesterol, promotes diuresis, and is cytotoxic particularly to colon cancer cells, antibacterial, antiviral, antiparasitic, and promotes healing of all tissues and prevents clots by thinning the blood through decreased platelet aggregation. One teaspoon of raw ginger steeped in hot water for ten minutes is my preferred route of administration.[68a, b]

Ginkgo biloba from the leaves of the ancient Chinese tree contains ginkosides, papaverine, flavonoids, flavone glycosides, terpene lactones, and many other phytochemicals with strong antioxidant activity that increases blood flow through small vessels such as in the brain, allowing for increases in oxygen uptake. Theoretically, this should improve blood flow to the optic nerve in glaucoma, and cognitive function and memory in dementia, asthma, coronary artery disease, depression, tinnitus of vascular origin, menopause, peripheral arterial disease, and age-related macular degeneration. Research studies have varied between denying its effectiveness and touting its results. It can be taken as a tea or capsule at a recommended dose of 40 mg three times daily and increase gradually for maximum effect.[69]

Ginseng (*panax ginseng*) root extract is the classic adaptogen for renewal of vigor, extension of stamina, regulation of hormones, and full function of the immune system. Its ginsenosides, polysaccharides, saponins, gintonins, and glycosyltransferases show powerful stimulation activities for treatment of depression, ADHD, erectile dysfunction and fatigue, prevention of stroke, memory loss, and other neurodegenerative disorders, and cytotoxic activities against microbes and cancer. Average recommended dosage is 2 to 4 grams a day. Note that ginseng includes a family of plants with slightly different properties. American ginseng (*panax quinquefolius*) is good for fatigue and possible stamina in sexual performance. Red Korean ginseng is a general energizer and good metabolic regulator. The other ginsengs are different plants altogether (Indian, Siberian, and Brazilian).[70]

Glucosamine/chondroitin is a nutraceutical combination that has been shown to be effective in the treatment of knee osteoarthritis and relief of symptomatic spinal disc degeneration, particularly at an early stage. It has beneficial effects on cells derived from synovial joints, knee, elbow, etc. by increasing type II collagen and proteoglycan formation, reducing inflammatory mediators and reducing cell death. Though more clinical trials are demanded and closely scrutinized, an average dosage of 1,500 mg a day appears to give effective relief in many cases. International societies are more supportive of its use.

(At age forty, my own racquetball-injured knee cartilage healed completely after six weeks of treatment, despite the surgery recommendation.[71 a, b])

Goatweed (*Capraria biflora* and *C. dulcis*) appears to be a relative of the Mexican pazote plants all containing varying amounts of betulinic acid + 1,4-0-naphthoquinone (biflorin) which are cytotoxic to bacteria and cancer cells. Known as "the pays" in the French West Indies, the leaves also contain sesquiterpenes, acopaudulin, which are active against viruses, and also ricin oil which makes it toxic in high doses. (A 1.8 mg dose of ricin, the size of a few grains of rice, is lethal to the average human.) It is used for digestive problems, blood purification, wound healing, conjunctivitis treatment, inflammation, and as a prevention of cancer. It is taken as one to two dried leaves in a tea, dosage unknown.[72]

*Goji berry (*Lycium barbarum*) is an exotic fruit with very powerful antioxidant activity, which enables it to affect cancer cells, prevent and reduce inflammation, boost the immune system, regulate blood pressure, reduce stress and anxiety, and reduce blood sugar levels in type 2 diabetes. It contains very high levels of vitamin C (ascorbic acid), vitamin A (betacarotene), the B vitamins, polysaccharides, trace elements and minerals and eighteen amino acids. Fresh fruit is the most effective method of consumption

as dried berries contain less vitamin C. Caution: too much vitamin C may cause diarrhea, and it should be avoided in pregnancy as it tends to cause uterine contractions.[73a, b]

Goldenseal (*Hydrastis canadiensis*) contains the proven antibacterial alkaloids, berberine, and hydrastine, which prevent the adherence of bacteria to cell mucosal walls in both the renal and gastric systems to treat inflamed intestines and urinary bladder infections. It is very effective in the treatment of sore throat and earaches, as one drop of tincture in a half cup of warm water. As an antibiotic it is effective against gonorrheal organisms.[74]

Gooseberry (*Philanthus acidus*) contains high levels of antioxidant anthocyanins, vitamins, and minerals that are effective against several conditions. The leaves can be used for sciatica, seeds as a cathartic in gastric problems, the roots as a purgative, the fruit as a gastric juices and blood enhancer. Recent studies confirm its effect against cancer cells.[75a, b]

Gotu kola (*Centella asiatica*) is a pennywort native of the Himalayan mountains. Containing high levels of terpenoid saponins, it reduces excessive scar tissue formation by inhibiting the overproduction of collagen. It can be used to assist in wound healing after surgery, to prevent cellulite and to strengthen valves in the veins. As a nervine, it improves blood circulation in the brain.[76]

Grapefruit (*Citrus paradisi*) contains citronellal, linalool, limonene, pectin, fiber, flavonoids, potassium, naringenin, and naringin, which help promote a healthy heart, reduce risk of ischemic stroke, and help with weight loss, mainly by reducing blood lipid levels, improving glucose intolerance and suppressing liver production of glucose. With its high water content, it counteracts dehydration and helps to maintain skin health. Caution: excess intake may interfere with hypertension medications as well as effects of antidepressants, quinine, and cyclosporine as it increases potassium levels.[77a, b]

Grapeseed extract (*Vitis vinifera*) mainly from dark muscadine grapes, contains high levels of flavanols, like resveratrol, with antioxidant activity that reduces the risk of vascular disease by regulation of platelet activity and reduction of red blood cell adhesions. It has proanthocyanidins, which protect the human lens epithelium from oxidative stresses associated with cataract formation, and vitamins and mineral for heart and skin health. The dosage of four to six glasses would be too high to involve red wine on a daily basis.[78a, b]

*Graviola *(Annona muricata)* or soursop contains the anticancer alkaloid, annonacin, in the fruit and acetogenins in the leaf, fruit, seeds, stem, and bark, which kill virus-like cancer cells without harming healthy cells. They are effective in very low doses against lung, breast, prostate, pancreas, colon, and liver carcinomas and adenocarcinomas. It has been known to kill bacteria, parasites, and viruses in addition to its more pleasant stimulation of digestion and relief of depression and insomnia, especially when consumed as ice cream or as a tea. Caution: too much annonacin or regular intake in hypersensitive individuals can cause Parkinson-like movements, temporary paralysis of eye muscles, and may induce premature labor in pregnancy.[79a, b]

Green tea (*Camellia sinensis*) is one of the super plants. With epigallocatechins and polyphenolic compounds, it kills existing tumor cells, imparts protection against the development of cancer and promotes the formation and excretion of metabolites of carcinogens. With only 0.3% caffeine, it is the non-oxidized form of tea. Its mechanisms of action include inhibition of the interaction of estrogens and their receptors, anti-proliferation of cancer cells, anti-inflammation and strong antioxidant free radical scavenging. It is used for cancer, inflammation, and infection protection of all organ systems, weight loss through metabolism regulation, blood pressure regulation, lowering cholesterol levels, prevention of tooth decay, and inhibition of blood clots. One cup daily is recommended for prevention and reduction of excess caffeine dependency, and four cups daily for existing cancer.[80a, b]

Guava *(Psidium guajava)* contains high levels of the antioxidants, caryophyllene, lycopene, nerol, quercetin, vitamin C, various tannins, and lots of fiber. As an antibiotic, it ruptures bacterial cell walls and membranes. Extracts of guava are cancer protective and act as an effective control of diarrhea associated with microbial infections. It is also useful against malaria resistant to conventional medications.[81]

Guggul (*Commiphora wightii*) resin is widely used in Asia as a cholesterol-lowering agent. It contains guggulsterones which may antagonize hormone receptors in cholesterol metabolism. Large scale studies have been scarce but effective use has been reported.[82]

Hawthorn berry (*Crataegus monogyna* and *laevgata* +) is a group of red berries high in flavonoids like vitexin, rutin, and quercetin, proanthocyanidins like epicatechin and procyanidin, triterpene acids like ursolic, oleanolic and crataegolic, and tannins. Through their antioxidant action, they aid digestion and regulate cardiovascular functions by improving exercise tolerance and reducing dyspnea and fatigue. Used to prevent and treat congestive heart failure and arrhythmic cardiac conditions, the recommended dosage ranges from 160 to 900mg a day.[83a, b]

Hesperidin is a flavone glycoside found in citrus fruit whose activity is largely cardiovascular in protecting blood vessels from harmful free radicals (immune system), maintaining lipid levels (metabolic), and neuroprotection. When exposed to the enzyme glucosidase and water, it produces hesperetin and rutinose which are the active ingredients. It is used to improve poor blood circulation in the lower extremities, heal leg ulcers and reduce hemorrhoids. The recommended dosage varies between

150 and 500 mg daily together with butcher's broom and vitamin C.[84a, b]

Hibiscus (*H. sabdariffa*) contains high levels of flavonoids like hibiscetin, delphinidol and cyanidinol, citric and malic acids, glucosides and anthrocyanins, which act to lower blood pressure by blocking the ACE inhibitors in the blood at the level of the kidneys. Triterpenoids block cancer cell migration in the breast and induce cell death (apoptosis). Hibiscus teas are effective in lowering cholesterol and blood sugar, liver protection, and as an antibiotic particularly against E. coli, proteus, and streptococcus infections.[85a, b]

*****Honey** made by bees of the genus apis consists mainly of the monosaccharides, fructose, and glucose. In a supersaturated liquid form. Methylglyoxal is the component of Manuka honey from the *Leptospermum scoparium* flower that has been shown to have antibiotic properties against some forms of MRSA (methicillin resistant staphylococcus aureus) in animal studies. Wound treatments with honey have been inconclusive. When used with hot water it has been known to soothe the sore throat.[86a, b]

Honeysuckle (*Lonicera periclymenum*) contains flavonoids, saponins, phenolics like chlorogenic and caffeic acids, luteolins, and the anti-inflammatory, loniceroside, which seeks to achieve vascular homeostasis through inhibition of platelet aggregation (prevents blood clotting). When used to treat influenza, it reduces the symptoms of fever, headaches, cough and sore throat. Its lignan component, hydnocarpin, suppresses the proliferation of colon and lung cancer cells.[87a, b]

Hops (*Humulus lupulus*) contain flavonoids and prenylflavonoids like xanthohumol, which through anti-proliferative activities of inhibition of aromatase have been shown to reduce breast, renal, and prostate cancer cells. As a potent phytoestrogen, it relieves the symptoms of menopause, especially hot flashes. Daily intake of four to six ounces is recommended.[88a, b]

Horsechestnut (*Aesculus hippocastanum*) with natural rutosides has traditionally been used to prevent blood clots following surgeries and reduction of edema due to chronic venous insufficiency in the lower extremities. A dosage of 300 mg along with elastic compression stockings at 20 to 30 mmHg at the ankle have been shown to be effective in preventing thrombosis events.[89a, b]

Horseradish (*Cochlearia armoracia*) is a natural antibiotic with mucosal irritants as effective for sinusitis as synthetic drugs. Containing sinipin, glucosinolates, allylisothiocyanates, and vitamin C, it is a rubefacient which increases the blood circulation to the face, promotes mucus expulsion from the sinuses, acts as a gastric stimulant and has some diuretic activity. The recommended dosage for acute colds and respiratory infections is 20 grams daily of fresh root. Caution: should be used in the presence of stomach ulcers and kidney ailments as well as in pregnancy as it may stimulate uterine contractions.[90]

Horsetail (*Equisetum arvense*) contains silicon, oxalic acid, and calcium oxalate, ingredients of bone, and so has been recommended for bone health. However, research studies uphold its use in the treatment of inflammatory disorders, associated with wound healing, bleeding, and ulcerations more than with bone health. Caution as some preparations contain thiaminase which may induce edema and loss of motor control leading to falls, nicotine, and may cause slowed heart rate and irregular heart rhythms. [91]

Inula (*I. racemosa)* is an alpine sunflower plant with adrenergic beta-blocking properties (vasodilation) that are cardioprotective, reduce anxiety, lowers cholesterol and blood sugar levels. It may be used to treat ischemic heart disease and respiratory diseases like asthma and bronchitis. Containing eudesmane, terpenoids, and essential oils, with antiseptic and disinfectant properties, it is an effective antibiotic, anti-inflamatory, and antiallergic tonic.[92]

Jaborandi (*Pilocarpus pennatifolius*) is a source of the parasympathomimetic alkaloid, pilocarpine, best known for its use in treating glaucoma, by constriction of the pupil and increase in aqueous outflow capacity. It is used in tablet form to treat dry mouth due to radiation and dry eyes due to Sjogren's syndrome. It causes sweating (diaphoresis) and is used to treat diarrhea.[93]

Jasmine (*Jasminium grandiflorum*) contains the lipid-based hormone, methyl jasmonate, which produces a vasorelaxant effect through the release of nitric oxide and activation of potassium to release calcium from the constricted cell. It is most often used as a tea for relaxation in conditions of stress.[94]

Jatoba (*Hymenaea courbacil*) is a large tropical tree whose resinous sap contains anti-inflammatory phytic acids and astringent tannins that can treat prostatitis and reduce diarrhea and excessive menstrual discharge. It has terpenes and phenolics that have antifungal, anti-yeast, and antitumor properties effective against Candida, athlete's foot and other yeast infections.[95]

Juana la blanca (*Borreria laevis*) is a ubiquitous plant on Puerto Rico, containing alkaloids, iridoids, flavonoids, terpenoids, and lots of iron. It has strong anti-inflammatory and antioxidant properties, which are effective in early cancer and dissolution of kidney stones. Usually taken as a tea, its relaxation of smooth muscles and diuresis make effective in reducing high blood pressure.[96]

Juniper berry (*Juniperus communis*) is the cone of the female conifer and not a true berry. Its oil has pinenes, which act as a diuretic, antibacterial, and antiseptic for problems of the urinary tract. By promoting appetite from the release of insulin from the pancreas, it is used mainly in northern European cuisine as a spice and to flavor gin.[97]

Kava kava (*Piper methysticum*) contains kavalactones, which show sedation, anticonvulsive, local anesthetic, and neuroprotective properties through muscle relaxation and a GABA-like reduction of brain waves in cases of mild to moderate stress-related anxiety, restlessness, and insomnia. Available as a tea, powder and tincture, it is used throughout the South Pacific islands for ritual and relaxation purposes. Overuse may reduce its effect and it should be avoided together with alcohol and other sedation drugs.[98]

Kutaki (*Picorrhiza kurroa*) root has a long history of use for digestive problems, but appears to be effective for the treatment of vitiligo when taken by mouth. Although it shows antioxidant, anti-inflammatory, and immunomodulatory activities with its luteolin and picein contents, it is most effective as a hepatoprotective (liver protection) agent.[99]

Lecithin is a phospholipid found in foods like egg yolks and organ meats, which releases choline and inositol to produce acetylcholine that helps the nerve cells in learning, memory, and cardiac function. It is usually taken as a supplement. Too much lecithin may be linked to production of a harmful chemical, TMAO, by gut bacteria that may actually contribute to heart disease.[100]

*__Legumes__ are low glycemic index foods like beans, peas, chickpeas, and hummus. They contain protease inhibitors that improve diabetic glucose tolerance, reduce the risk of heart disease and cancer, and also reduce the level of total cholesterol. They also contain high amounts of isoflavone antioxidants and fiber.[101]

*__Lemon__ (*Citrus limon/ C. major*) is one of the wonder fruit that has potent antiseptic, disinfectant, antibacterial, and antioxidant activity against infections in practically all organ systems. Containing citric acid, high levels of vitamin C, citroene, limonene, hesperetin, naringen, and several terpenes, it is an effective aid to digestion and liver detoxification.[102]

Lemonbalm (*Melissa officinalis*) contains citrals, citronella, citronello, flavonoids, rosmarinic acid, and phenols whose antioxidant action disrupts the cell walls of cancer cells, aids digestion, confers analgesia, mild sedation, and heals herpes sores by blocking the virus entry into skin cells. May be taken as a tea, or an extract, and also in a skin cream for Alzheimer's, colon cancer, and herpes simplex sores.[103 a, b]

Lemongrass (*Cymbopogon citratus*) contains citrals, citronella, and terpenes, which make cancer cells self-destruct through apoptosis, suppress COX-2 expression against inflammation, is antispasmodic and extends relaxation. It is effective against herpes simplex, antibacterial, antifungal, relieves arthritis, and aids digestion. (*Lemon verbena officinalis and Melissa officinalis have similar properties.*)[104 a, b]

Licorice (*Glycyrrhia glabra*) contains flavonoids, glycyrrhizin, deoxyglycyrrhetol, and glycyrrhetinic acid, which are active against HIV, HSV, and influenza viruses of lungs and liver and gastrointestinal tract. Through its antioxidant activity, it is very effective against GERD and helps with healing existing stomach ulcers. Caution: excess intake may deplete potassium levels and result in increased blood pressure. An effective dosage is two tablespoons of deglycerrhized licorice root at bedtime.[105]

Life plant (*Kalanchoe pinnata*) bufadienolides, coumarinic, behenic, and caffeic acids, mucilages, strong antioxidants, and alkaloids, which act against bacteria, viruses, and fungi to promote wound healing in cases of injury and skin ulcers, inflammation, and pain reduction, and relief of cold and flu symptoms. The leaves are heated to extract the essential oils, which can be applied topically or taken as an infusion of one cup of 1 to 2 grams daily. It can be toxic if overdosed.[106]

Lobelia (*L. inflata*) is also known as "Indian tobacco" and was smoked by Native Americans as a treatment for asthma and other respiratory conditions. Though its main ingredient is lobeline, which is competitive with nicotine for receptors, it was found to be ineffective as a substitute for conventional cigarette addiction and somewhat effective for asthma when taken in very small doses of less than 0.1 grams. Caution: as an overdose, this is toxic and may cause nausea, vomiting, dizziness, diarrhea, heart palpitations, and decreased blood pressure. It is a smooth muscle relaxant.[107]

*Lutein (along with zeaxanthin and azaxanthin) is a carotenoid found in dark, leafy vegetables and eggs, which is a prominent pigment in the macula of the eye and responsible for lower risk of chronic age-related eye diseases like macular degeneration and cataracts. It is believed to act as a protective filter against harmful ultraviolet radiation and antioxidant against cataracts formed from oxidative stress. The daily recommended intake is from 20 to 40 mg, which is more effective as whole food than in supplement form.[108]

*Lycopene, a carotenoid in cooked tomatoes, has been associated with a reduced risk of lethal prostate and found to reduce PSA levels and the swelling of benign prostate hyperplasia (BPH). For its antioxidant action dosages of 50 to 75mg daily in capsule or softgel form for six to eight weeks have been deemed effective. For prevention, a cup of cooked tomatoes or sauce three to four times a week may be effective. Caution: as tomato-based products are acidic and may promote and irritate stomach ulcers.[109a, b]

Maca root (*Lepidium meyenii*) is a Peruvian root tuber that contains many phytochemicals including amino and fatty acids, carbohydrates, fats and proteins, sterols, high in iron, magnesium, selenium, and calcium, has been touted as an aphrodisiac especially for sexual dysfunction on menopausal women. It is an effective energizer, booster of stamina and nutritional health adjunct with antioxidant properties and healing action. A few studies have upheld its claim to counteract depression in menopausal women and reduce fatigue in elderly men. A positive effect on human endocannabinoid receptors through its N-alkylamides and acylethanolamine signaling system has been established, which supports its anti-stress and somewhat euphoric properties. Its enhancement of luteinizing hormones in female rats supports its use to promote fertility. Though available as a powder, it is most effective in its natural root form, eaten raw or cooked.[110a, b]

Mace (*Myristica fragans*) has a strong free radical scavenging antioxidant activity (second of the spices behind cloves), which is beneficial to human health. It displays high-binding activity to the cannabinoid receptor CB1 and as such may result in somewhat similar reactions of euphoric "high." It has a positive effect on digestion through the cytochrome P450 system as well as mild to moderate anti inflammation properties.[111a, b]

Magnesium deficiency can result from stress. Among the approximately three hundred metabolic processes requiring magnesium, it is needed for the proper transport of calcium across cell membranes. Insufficiency can lead to calcium buildup in arterial vessels then stroke and cardiac arrest. As an anti-inflammatory mineral, it is used to remedy high blood pressure, arthritis, respiratory diseases, ADD, age-related macular degeneration, migraine, osteoporosis, constipation, insomnia, and diabetes. Found in almonds, cashews, peanuts, pumpkin seeds, kidney beans, spinach, halibut, avocado, and dark chocolate, the RDA daily requirement is estimated to be between 240 to 420 mg depending on age. Magnesium L-Threonate is a good supplement for mental clarity and focus.[112]

Maiden apple (*Momordica charantia*), also known as cundeamor and bitter melon, is a climbing vine with orange spiky fruit with sweet tasting red seeds. Hailed as a cure for diabetes, studies are currently underway to determine an effective dosage and possible side effects. The hypoglycemic effects of charantin has potential for lowering blood sugar levels by increasing insulin sensitivity but has not been firmly established when compared to conventional medications.[113]

Mango (*Mangifera indica*) contributes dried flowers with tannins for relief of diarrhea, ripe fruit with mangiferin, mangiferol, and high levels of vitamin C, green fruit and resin with acids as antibiotics for scabies, bark with mangiferine for rheumatism and asthma and leaves with glucosides for diabetes and hypertension. In addition, there are phenolics, flavonols, and terpenoids, which have anticancer and antibacterial properties through antioxidant activity. Caution: burning the wood is a toxic irritant, the fruit containing high levels of fructose and sucrose may raise the blood sugar to dangerous levels in diabetics, and some people are extremely hypersensitive to the sap of the fruit rind. Eating one mango a day during season is a fairly safe regimen.[114]

Marjoram (*Origanum majorana*) is used primarily as a culinary in preparing soups, stews, sauces, and meat dishes. With the anti-inflammation activity of its essential oils, it aids the digestive processes to prevent gastritis, protects the gastrointestinal walls from excess acid and harmful bacteria, and relieves both diarrhea and constipation. As a vasodilator, it enhances the cardiovascular system by lowering blood pressure and reducing cholesterol. Some of its active chemicals are borneol, camphor, quercetin, jaceidin, and pinene. Two tablespoon of marjoram is loaded with antioxidants, vitamins, minerals, and other phytonutrients.[115]

Marshmallow root is a major natural product for the prevention and treatment of sore throat, mouth and gastric ulcers, through its soothing action on mucous membranes. With high levels of mucilages like altheahexacosanyl lactone, calamenes, coumarin glucosides, lauric acid, beta-sitosterol and lanosterol, in the leaves, flowers, and root; it also has lipid lowering and platelet aggregation properties to prevent blood clotting and cardiovascular accidents as well as antimicrobial potential.[116]

Melatonin (N-acetyl-5-methoxy tryptamine) is a pineal gland hormone directly derived from the amino acid, tryptophan, a precursor for serotonin, a "feel good" neurotransmitter. It signals sleep time in accordance with the arrival of darkness, regulates reactions to changes in daylight and darkness, appropriate blood pressure, and acts as a powerful antioxidant protector of nuclear and mitochondrial DNA. It can be used as a sleep aid and in the treatment of some sleep disorders. Though cherries are a good natural source, it can be taken orally as capsules, tablets, or liquids, sublingually or as a transdermal patch. As natural levels decrease with age, the ensuing insomnia may be offset be resetting the biorhythms with a dose of 1 to 10mg usually one hour before bedtime. It is an excellent sleep aid for air travel in an eastward direction. Recent studies indicate that melatonin may have positive activity against cancer cell growth.[117 a, b]

Milk thistle (*Silybum marianum*) lowers cholesterol; prevents and treats liver problems like cirrhosis, jaundice, hepatitis, and gall bladder disorders; and benefits diabetes, through the antioxidant and anti inflammatory activities of silymarin, flavonoids, phenolic acids, and flavolignans. It has shown positive effects on liver function in alcohol related liver disease when given as Liverubin in one study. By enhancing hepatocyte protein synthesis in the liver, it can replace and repair damaged liver tissue and serve as protection during chemotherapy. The average daily intake for protection is 175 mg a day, while higher dosages may be needed for repair.[118a, b]

Mimosa (*M. pudica*) contains the toxic alkaloid "mimosine" as well as the psychoactive dimethyltryptamine (DMT) which in addition to their hallucinogenic properties, show antiproliferative and apoptotic action in killing the larvae of the some intestinal worms. These phytochemicals can neutralize cobra venom by inhibiting its enzymatic activity. It may be used as a substrate for psychotria viridis, one of the ingredients in the ayahuasca brew. It contains several hydroxyflavanones which exhibit strong anti-inflammation activity. Its tiny leaves fold inwards when touched as a defense against harm and unfold a few minutes later.[119]

*__Moringa__ (*M. oleifera*) is known as the tree of life due to the abundance and variety of ingredients in its leaves, flowers, stems, and roots. Uniquely, it contains moringa YSP, niazimicin, and zeatin, which are immunomodulatory and kill toxic to cancer cells. In addition it has kaempferol, eighteen amino acids, thirty-six anti-inflammatories, chlorophyll, omega 3 and 6, and many other phytonutrients, vitamins, and minerals. It is used as a natural energy booster, internal and external healing agent, Alzheimer's prevention by its promotion of cholinergic and antioxidant activity, anti-inflammatory, diuretic for high blood pressure, immunity booster, digestive aid, blood sugar regulator for diabetes, kidney regulator, antibacterial, antiviral, antifungal, and skin rejuvenator. The recommended dosage is one teaspoon of dried leaves in salad, added to rice, eggs, stew, soups, sauces, or tea daily for treatment and weekly for prevention. Caution should be used in not taking too much or during pregnancy as it thickens the blood.[120 a, b]

__MSM__ (*methylsulfonylmethane*) is an organosulfur compound that has potent antioxidant and anti-inflammation activities especially effective in the treatment of arthritis by inhibiting the enzymes that block nitric oxide therefore allowing more to be available for regulation of the inflammatory process as well as inhibiting the viability of inflammation cells. It is especially effective in reducing the pain of osteoarthritis. A recommended supplemental dosage is between 2000 to 6000mg daily with meals or 1000mg orally three times a day.[121]

Mullein (*Verbascum thapsus*) contains mucilages (harpagoside, laterioside, glucopyranoside), which soothe and heal irritated mucous membranes. It is used most often for ear infections of both viral and bacterial origins, as well as treating hemorrhoids, worms, and immediate relief in some asthma attacks. Its kaempferol content is effective against inflammatory lung and gastric conditions. Made from its dried leaves and flowers, it may be taken as a juice, tea, oil, or tincture.[122]

Mumefural (*Prunus mume*) or Japanese plum (more closely related to an apricot) contains a citric acid derivative, flavonoids, and natural phytonutrients used to improve blood flow and as a tonic for natural purification of the blood and to promote liver and immune system health. Its antibiotic resinols inhibit the bacteria Helicobactor pylori in gastritis and stomach ulcers as well as prevention and treatment of dental diseases associated with bacteria. It enhances the oxidative capacity of exercising skeletal muscle enabling it to use fatty acids as fuel instead of carbohydrates, thereby promoting endurance. It is available pickled, as plum juice, wine, or as dried herbal tea.[123a, b]

*Mushrooms (Maitake *(Grifola frondosa)*, *Shiitake (Lentinula edodes) and Reischii (Ganoderma lucidum)*) all have potent antioxidant properties that help to prevent and

treat infections, inflammations, and the general wear and tear of ageing, largely through their enhancement of the immune system response. Maitake is used to stimulate the immune system cells in breast cancer patients and has a portion known as Maitake D-fraction, which appears to reduce the risk of metastasis. With its alpha-glucosidase inhibitors, it has a hypoglycemic effect on diabetic patients. Its antioxidants inhibit angiogenesis by reducing VEGF (vascular endothelial growth factor) to prevent abnormal new blood vessel formation and subsequent excessive spontaneous bleeding. Shiitake is used more as a food nutrient but has healing properties owing to its high content of vitamins and minerals. Reischii is used during cancer chemotherapy to boost the immune system function as well as for its anti-inflammation effects on allergies like asthma and contact dermatitis. With an abundance of antibiotics, antioxidants, cholesterol inhibitors, immunosuppressants, and immunostimulants, all three are found on the routine treatment regimens at the Sloan Kettering Cancer Center in NYC.[124 a, b, c]

Myrrh (*Commiphora myrrha*) is a natural resin of a gum tree. Its essential oil is an oleoresin, traditionally used as a perfume, incense, and medicine. When mixed in wine (alcohol extract), it can be ingested to improve blood circulation, problems of arthritis, and menopausal irregularities. It can be found in mouthwashes, gargles, and toothpastes for its analgesia and the prevention and treatment of gum disease. It is also known to reduce (LDL) cholesterol and raise the HDL, as well as reduce blood glucose levels.[125a, b]

Natto is a traditional Japanese food made from soybeans fermented with Bacillus subtilis or B. natto bacteria. It contains the specific enzyme, nattokinase, a serine protease, which along with several nattozimes, exhibits fibrinolytic activity (prevents and breaks up blood clots) and strongly promotes blood circulation and cardiovascular health.[126]

Neem (*Azadirachta indica*) trees contain azadiratin, triperpenoids, steroids, acids, and triglycerides which give it antiseptic, antibacterial, antiviral, antifungal, antiparasitic, and anticancer properties. It is used in soaps, disinfectants, toothpaste, shampoos, anti-itch creams, and liniments. It is effective against psoriasis, eczema, and dermatitis. As a natural pesticide, it is very effective against mosquitoes and other pesky insects.[127]

Nettles (*Urtica dioica*), of which stinging nettle is a prototype, is used for the relief of the acute allergic reaction and chronic allergies from contact with the histaminic trichromes in the leaves of the plant. The leaves that dealt the poison also contain the remedy in its acetylcholine, morodin, and anti-histaminic leukotrienes that counteract the reacton by inhibiting TNF-alpha and cytoknes. Taken orally, it relieves allergic rhinitis and promotes health function of the prostate and urinary tract systems.[128]

Noni (*Morinda citrifolia*) contains parafin, acids, alcohols, polysaccharides, anthraquinones, vitamins, minerals, lignans, and special phytochemicals, xeronine, and morindin, which give it strong antiparasitic and antiinflammation properties. Used as a detoxification agent, it is also a natural pesticide against worms, shows preventive activity against colon cancer and dental caries. It is available in juice, capsules, and powders. *Caution* should be exercised in cases of liver and kidney disorders, as it contains high levels of potassium and large amounts may be toxic.[129]

*****Nuts** , like cashew, contain essential oils that kill bacteria and fungi and are effective in relief of diarrhea and fever. Walnuts contain phenolics like ferulic acid and myricetin, with the highest rating for antioxidants. Almonds with aflatoxin contamination from molds are carcinogenic until pasteurized, then their oils are rich in monounsaturated fats like oleic and linoleic acids and vitamin E for skin health. Pistachios contain palmitic and stearic fatty acids, carbohydrates, proteins, carotenoids, vitamins, and minerals. A handful of nuts daily contributes to general health and well being.[130a, b, c]

Oatmeal and bran, whole grains and fiber, improve digestive tract function like prevention of constipation, reduction of pain of irritable bowel syndrome, prevent colon and breast cancer, lower cholesterol levels, regulate glucose metabolism and lower blood pressure, through its high content of insoluble fiber. The effective recommended dosage for GI tract functions is 20 to 25 grams per day and for blood pressure and cholesterol is 6 to 10 grams per day.[131a, b]

*Olive (*Olea europa*) oil of the fruit and leaf of the tree are both intensely medicinal. Cold pressed extra virgin olive oil, loaded with omega 3 fatty acids, vitamins, minerals, protein, phytosterols, mono and polyunsaturated fats and saturated fats, is preferred. Tyrosol and hydroxytyrosol strengthen blood vessel walls, regulate platelets to reduce clumping and increase bone formation. Oleic acid lowers LDL cholesterol, which protects the heart and cardiovascular system. Other polyphenols and antioxidants decrease the production of messaging molecules and decrease oxidative stress for cancer protection. Ligostride inhibits the growth of Heliobacter pylori bacteria in the gut and aids digestion. The average dosage is three (3) tablespoons a day.[132]

Omega 3 polyunsaturated fatty acids include DHA (docosahexaenoic acid, found in the retina), EPA (eicosapentaenoic acid, for cell membrane integrity, blood clotting and blood pressure), ALA (alpha linolenic acid, for cognitive health like Alzheimer's), and GLA (gamma linolenic acid, for reduction of joint inflammation and pain) and others. All have antioxidant, anti-inflammatory, anti-clotting, neuro-protective, anticancer, antidepressant, and heart health properties. The recommended preventive dosage is 1000mg supplement per day or two servings of oily cold water fish per week.[133a, b]

Onions (*Allium cepa*) are a primary source of quercetin, biotin, manganese, vitamin B1, B6, C and folate, copper, phosphorus, potassium and fiber. They help reduce the risk of Parkinson's disease, heart disease, stroke, and inflammation. Their cysteine sulfoxides, flavonoids, disulfides, trisulfides, capaene, and vinyldithins have strong antioxidant, antimicrobial and anticancer properties. Folate helps to make new cells. Quercetin helps to reduce plaques in arteries, relax airway muscles in asthma and reduce allergic reactions by blocking antihistamine production. Daily consumption in menopause improves bone density and reduces the risk of osteoporosis in menopause. *Caution* as they contain vitamin K and may enhance the action of blood thinners. One medium onion a day will give all around benefits.[134a, b]

Oregano (*Origanum vulgare*, etc.) herbs contain high concentrations of monoterpenes, acids like rosmarinic, oleanolic, and ursolic, and essential oils like carvacrol and thymol, which have active antibacterial, antioxidant, and anticancer properties. It is readily used in cuisine for flavoring grilled foods.[135]

Oysters (*Ostreidae* family) are mollusks with several unique nutrients and minerals, zinc, B vitamins, glycogen, omega 3 fatty acids, amino acids, and whose proposed aphrodisiac claims are most likely attributed to the stimulation of testosterone through HDL cholesterol enhancement and resulting improved blood circulation. They contribute to weight loss, tissue repair and growth, energy, reduction in blood pressure, improved immune system function, wound healing, and improved bone strength to reduce the risk of osteoporosis. Caution: raw oysters can harbor several harmful bacterial and parasitic pathogens as well as heavy metals and are not advised for consumption if pregnant.[136]

Oyster plant (*Rhoeo spathecea*) contain anthocyanins, phenolics, analgesics, and high levels of the antioxidant, vitamin E. Its rholanin is antibacterial, protective of small venous capillaries, and cytotoxic to cancer cells. It is used to treat skin eruptions and contusions, as well as respiratory conditions. Both decoctions and infusion teas are used.[137]

Papaya (*Carica p.*) contains the digestive enzymes, papain, carpain and chymotrypsin, pectin, alkaloids, fiber, vitamins, minerals, and glycosides in its leaves, fruit, seeds, latex sap, and roots. By breaking down heavy proteins, it is used as a meat tenderizer and digestive aid after fatty meals, antibacterial, and antihelminthic. Its antiinflammatory and immunomodulatory properties makes it cytotoxic to cancer cells, and its high levels of phytoestrogens reduce menopausal symptoms, especially vaginal dryness. A 780 mg serving of green papaya fruit with high potassium can reduce high blood pressure. Application of raw strips directly to a wound can assist healing. Caution: latex sap may be a toxic irritant to sensitive skin.[138]

Paprika is a spice made from air-dried fruit of red chili peppers (*Capsicum annum*) in which most of the seeds have been removed. Though chemically similar to cayenne pepper, it is not as hot. Used more for its culinary flavor, its color is due to xanthophyll carotenoid zeaxanthin. It still exhibits retains medicinal properties as an antibacterial agent and stimulant to normalize blood pressure, improve circulation and increase the production of saliva and gastric acids to help digestion. It has a very high level of vitamin C.[139]

Parsley (*Petroselenium crispum*) contains apiol oil, myristicin, coumarins, vitamins A, B and C, plus carbohydrates and fiber, which promote direct intestinal cleansing, hypertension control through diuresis, blood clot prevention through platelet aggregation, and blockage of cancer cell proliferation through inhibition of migration and antioxidant reduction of DNA damage.[140]

Passionflower (*Passiflora incarnata*) contains over 150 terpenoids, cyanogenic allocides, glucosides, high levels of vitamin C, which through its anti-inflammatory and antioxidant properties induces sedation by reducing nervous anxiety and insomnia. Its antioxidants and fiber lowers triglycerides and cholesterol by decreasing leptin and insulin. It also contains beta carboline alkaloids, which are hallucinogenic when smoked. It is most effective as an infusion tea taken at bedtime.[141]

Pau d'arco (*Tabebuia avellanedae or impetiginosa*) also known as lapacho contains lapachol, a strong antiviral against herpes simplex type 1 and 2 as well as colds and influenza. By inhibiting both the DNA and RNA polymerases and retrovirus reverse transcriptase to block proliferation and induce apoptosis (cell death) of cancer cells, it is effective against skin cancer, particularly squamous cell carcinoma.[142]

Peach (*Prunus persica*) is native to northwest China and is most valued for its nutritious fruit. In addition to antimicrobial properties, the leaves contain astringents that bind metabolites to create a state of constipation making it effective in counteracting diarrhea. The leaves of the guava and pigeon pea tees have a similar action.[143]

Peppermint (*Menta peperita*) contains phenobarbitol, atropine, menthol, eugenol, betaine, flavonoids, resins, and tannins that give it strong antiviral activity against herpes simplex type 1 and 2, as well as recurrent herpes. It is an appetite stimulant, digestive aid, antioxidant, antibacterial, sedative and respiratory aid through its decongestant actions. It is used to relieve the headache and congestion of sinusitis and discomfort of sore throat.[144]

Periwinkle *(Catharanthus roseus)* contains vinca indole alkaloids, the most effective of which are vincristine, vinpocetine, and vinblastine, which are cytotoxic to cancer cells by blocking mitosis reproduction through microtubule inhibition. Treatment is very effective against Hodgkin's lymphoma and certain leukemias. As more alkaloids are being isolated, additional properties like amoebicide, antibiotic, and analgesia are being found.[145a, b]

Persimmon (*Diospyros kaki*) is a berry-like tomato, high in glucose and low in protein. The skin contains malic acid, high fiber, vitamin C, and the important metabolic minerals, sodium, potassium, magnesium, calcium, iron, and manganese, plus pro-vitamin A beta-carotene, catechins, and betulinic acid, which are very active against cancer cells. Caution: eating the fruit on an empty stomach may cause "bezoars," which are hard wads of food that are virtually indigestible. These are often associated with the pesticides that are sprayed on the skin. Wash well.[146]

Picrorhiza kurroa is a Himalayan medicinal herb also known as *kutki*, with a history of use for digestive inflammation, asthma, viral hepatitis, and vitiligo. It contains apocynin that relieves inflammation by inhibiting the NADPH oxidase enzyme. Picroliv, a derivative reduces inflammation in gut tissue. The application of 200mg of powder twice a day in combination with oral methoxsalen may be beneficial to reducing the white skin patches of vitiligo. Its antioxidant, antiperoxidative activity on the myocardium may offers significant cardioprotective effects. The dosage and benefits for asthma due to respiratory allergy is in progress.[147a, b]

Pineapple (*Ananas comosus*) contains bromelain, a combination of two protease enzymes that process meat protein and reduce inflammation in the gut through its antioxidant, anti-inflammatory, and proteolytic activities. In addition, pineapple is high in fiber, vitamins (C and A), minerals especially manganese, folates, and coumarins, making it an effective blood thinner as well. The enzyme breaks down the proteins of parasites in the gut making it an effective anti-helminthic. Currently undergoing trials as a treatment for skin burns, it is effective in reducing the inflammation associated with allergic rhinitis, arthritis, indigestion and intestinal worms.[148a, b]

Plantain (*Plantago major*) also known as llantén, is a food medicine native to Europe and ubiquitous in the western tropics. Its active compounds include allantoin, flavonoids, aucubin, ursolic, citric, caffeic and oxalic acids, soothing mucilages, glucosides, coumarins, tannins, vitamins, minerals, gums, and resins, giving it a wide range of positive biological effects. It is used for healing gastric ulcers, replenishing nutrients lost in diarrhea, inflammation reduction, pain relief, and as an antibiotic, through its astringent, antioxidant, immune system regulating activities. Aucubin increases the uric acid excretion and may be useful in treating gout. A tea infusion of leaves and seeds is an effective method of dosing.[149]

Pomegranate (*Punica granatum*) is a fruit with a highest antioxidant ORAC ranking. It contains polyphenols, ellagitannins (punicalagins), granatin B, fatty acids, vitamin C, B complex vitamins, fiber, and minerals, which show strong anti-inflammatory and anti-proliferative activity in the prevention and treatment of prostate swelling (BPH) and cancer. Evidence exists for positive effects on breast cancer cells, lymphoma, and diabetic glucose levels.[150a, b, c]

*__Probiotics__ are fermented live bacteria that promote a healthy gut mucosal lining and have a positive effect on the digestion processes of inflammation reduction, diarrhea control, and intestinal infection. Useful bacteria include Lactobacillus acidophilus, L. rhamnosus, Saccharomyces boulardi, Streptococcus thermophiles, Bifidobacterium longum, and Lactococcus lactis. Ideally the ratio should be eighty-twenty with the beneficial bacteria predominant. This balance can be disrupted by stress, overuse of antibiotic medications, and poor diet. Improved digestion through changing the gut flora is a long-term process and must be accompanied by appropriate dietary changes and is well worth the effort. Dosages may contain from one to ten billion colony-forming-units (CFUs). An average probiotic dose would be one to two million CFUs three to four times a week, as tablets, liquids, or yogurt, and up to ten million CFUs daily to correct disorders for up to two weeks at a time.[151 a, b, c]

__Prunes__ (*Prunus domestica*) is a well-known commonly used product for the prevention and treatment of constipation. High in vitamins, minerals, sorbitol and fiber, its laxative action is related to the presence of antioxidant phenolics like chlorogenic and neochlorogenic acids, and oxyphenisatine. Effective dosages for prevention appear to be three to five prunes or one-half glass of juice, while twice the amount is needed plus increasing the amount of water intake to one to two quarts daily for relief of established constipation.[152]

Psyllium (*Plantago ovata*) is also known as ispaghula. The seed husk is a soluble fiber agent, which when added to water increases stool bulk and frequency for relief of constipation, but not as effective as prunes. It consists mainly of mucilage and dietary fiber. It is also useful for irritable bowel disease, diarrhea, reduction of glucose and cholesterol in type 2 diabetics, and reducing the risk of cardiovascular disease. It is available in capsules, and as one teaspoon in eight ounces of water one to two times a day as needed. It may also be used in gluten-free baking. Caution: choking may occur if taken with insufficient water.

Purslane (*Portulaca oleracea*), also known as verdalago, contains isoflavonoids, noradrenalin, cyanogenic glycosides, beta-sitosterol, vitamins, minerals, mucilages and highest level of omega 3 fatty acids of any vegetable. It may be used as an anti-inflammatory for sores, boils, diarrhea, hemorrhoids, as a hemostatic for intestinal and postpartum bleeding, as a detoxificaton agent for toxic chemicals like bisphenol A in plastics, is cytotoxic to several cancer cell lines and has been shown to improve glycemic and lipid status of type 2 diabetics. It may be eaten as a leaf vegetable, in salads, stir-fried, or cooked. Since it contains oxalates, cooking reduces the uric acid content.[154 a, b]

Quercetin is a flavonoid plant pigment found in fruit and vegetables like apples, grapes, berries, onions, broccoli, and buckwheat. Its inhibition of the release of histamine from mast cells in the blood and its antioxidant activity makes it useful in the prevention and treatment of allergic rhinitis, asthma, blood vessel integrity, obesity, and urticaria of the skin. Though the FDA is reluctant to grant it medicinal status based on inconclusive studies, the average dosage is between 1,000 to 1,500 mg a day for beneficial effects.[155a, b]

***Quinoa** (*Chenopodium quinoa*) is considered to be a "superfood." The seed grains have high-quality protein, essential amino acids, carbohydrates, fatty acids, fiber, vitamins, and minerals, and low in gluten. Its antioxidant activity make it effective in reducing inflammatory digestive issues, type 2 diabetes, hypertension control, prevention of colon cancer, weight loss for obesity, and when a complete whole grain protein is needed in place of animal protein. One cup twice to thice a week is nutritionally healthy.[156]

Raspberry leaf (*Rubus idaeus*) contains anthrocyanins, phenols, ellagitannins, and flavonoids effective for weight loss, female hormonal balance especially in second stage of labor, control of vomiting, through relaxation of blood vessels and regulation of basal metabolism.[157]

Red clover (*Trifolium pratense*) is one of the richest sources of the phytoestrogen, isoflavones, and is associated with women's health. Its antispasmodic, sedative, and anti-inflammatory actions are effective for menopausal hot flashes but caution should be exercised in pregnancy and in women with risk of estrogen-sensitive cancers. It may increase bone strength in osteoporosis.[158]

*Red wine (with resveratrol) is beneficial to obese individuals and diabetics by improving insulin sensitivity and lowering glucose production by activation of specific enzymes in the liver (much like metformin). The average recommended dosage for men is 8 oz /daily and for women, four ounces/daily. In most research studies, much higher dosages were required to get a significant effect; however, these dosages would bring secondary detrimental effects in humans.[159]

Red yeast rice is a whole grain fermented rice, which gets its color from being cultivated with the mold *Monascus purpureus* and, in addition to its culinary use, is best known for its ability to lower cholesterol, aid digestion, and purify the blood. Though its monacolin K chemical is identical to lovastatin, the statins are giant patented anticholesterol drugs while red yeast rice is a non-prescription dietary supplement on the back shelves. Both inhibit LDL cholesterol synthesis by blocking the enzyme HMG-CoA reductase. As controversy exists concerning the concentration of monacolin in the natural product, make sure it is from a reputable company and should be at least 10mg. The average dosage to lower cholesterol is 1,200mg twice a day. (160)

Rhodiola rosea is an arctic plant that contains over 140 phytochemicals including rhodionin, rosavin, rosin, rosarm, phenols,organic acids, terpenoids, flavonoids, anthraquinones,alkaloids,and essential oils.Used to improve mood and reduce anxiety, research confirms its positive effect on mild to moderate depression. The appropriate dose depends on age, health and nature of the condition.[161]

Rosemary (*Rosmarinus officinalis*) contains rosmarinic, ursolic, carnosic, and phenolic acids, camphor, papaverine, limonene, and many other terpenoids and sesquiterpenes, with strong antioxidant, antiseptic, hepatoprotective properties, and vasodilation to increase blood flow in small vessels. In addition to its culinary use, rosemary can decrease the risk of Alzheimer's and other dementias by maintaining blood flow to the brain and supporting enzymes necessary for cognition and learning. [162a, b, c]

Saffron (*Crocus sativus*) is a spice that contains the yellow carotenoids, picrocrocin, crocetin, and saffronal, the antioxidants,carsonic, turmeric, chlorogenic, and ursonic acids, which are anti-inflammatory, and help with digestion, asthma, cancer risk reduction, intraocular pressure control in glaucoma, and insomnia. An oral extract of 100mg a day is recommended for these conditions.[163a, b]

Safflower (*Carthamus tinctorius*) contains essential oils, vitamins, minerals, amino acids, and fatty acids like oleic (monounsaturated) and linolenic (polyunsaturated) that through its anti-inflammatory action, increases the protein, adiponectin, to regulate blood glucose and enable fatty acid breakdown. It can help with control in type 2 diabetes.[164]

Sage (*Salvia officinalis*) is a Mediterranean evergreen with culinary and medicinal uses. It contains the monoterpene, thujone, an ingredient of absinthe liquor, nicotinamide, flavones, tannins, and organic acids. Its antioxidant, antibiotic, cytotoxic and vascular enhancement activity makes it useful in the prevention and treatment of cancer, upper respiratory infections and cognitive dysfunction.[165]

Saltwater gargle is an efficient effective remedy for sore throat caused by virus or overuse of vocal cords. A warm gargle will increase blood flow to the area, encourage movement of mucus, reduce swelling by absorbing excess fluid from tissues, and relieve irritation and pain. One teaspoon salt dissolved in eight ounces of warm water used once an hour until relieved is the recommended regimen.

SAMe (S-adenosyl-L-methioine) ,a naturally occurring chemical compound of the body that repairs cartilage by increasing chondrocytes and lubricating joints, is effective in the treatment of some forms of osteoarthritis particularly the knee. Though it takes longer for results, there are fewer side effects than with the use of conventional anti inflammation drugs. It also increases levels of serotonin and dopamine in the central nervous system (CNS) and is used to treat depression. An effective dose is between 250 to 500mg twice a day.[166a, b]

Sarsaparilla (*Smilax ornata*) root was traditonally used to treat syphilis. Its saponins and flavonoids have antioxidant, anti-inflammation and antifungal properties with benefits to autoimmune diseases. It is available as teas, drinks, capsules and tinctures.[167]

Sassafras (*S. albicans*) contains safrole, anethole, pinene, camphor, eugenol and myristicin with COX 2 inhibition anti-inflammation actions like the NSAIDS and cytotoxic activity through induced DNA breaks in cancer cells.[168]

Saw palmetto (*Serenoa repens*) from the date berries of the palm contains flavonoids, phytosterols and fatty acids that help to prevent and reduce early prostatic swelling (BPH) by inhibiting the hormone dihydrotestosterone (DHT), which influences prostate size and reducing inflammation, which causes swelling. The reduction in size allows for easier urinary flow. Apparently the compound has little or no effect on cancer prevention or cure. Effective dose is around 160mg daily.[169]

Schizandra (*S. chinensis*)seed oil contains schizandrin, gomisin, and fatty acids with strong antioxidant, sedative, and hypnotic activity. It is used for stress-related conditions like anxiety and depression. Effective recommended dose is 500 mg daily.[170]

*Seaweed** with nutritional and medicinal value can be brown (kelp, wakame), green (algae, dulse, seagrass, spirulina, chlorella, dashi), and red (nori). They contain varying amounts of iodine, fiber, proteins, like alginate, agar and carrageenan, and polysaccharides. Their specific and combined actions stimulate gut enzymes to breakdown and absorb large proteins and complex molecules. They appear to be beneficial in the prevention of cancer associated with viruses. They are effective in metabolic support in the treatment of thyroid cancer and detoxification of heavy metals. When added to water, they assist with the removal of undesired elements like nitrites, nitrates, ammonium, phosphates, iron, copper and carbon dioxide. Kelp contains a sulfated polysaccharide, fucoidan, which stimulates the immune system to regulate inflammation and kill cancer cells. They all help to boost the immune system. The recommended intake is several tablets or fresh cooked, especially accompanying the ingestion of possibly contaminated fish.[171]

*Selenium disulfide (SeS2) is an inorganic compound with strong antioxidant activity in protection of cell membranes from free radicals. It is antifungal for the topical treatment of seborrheic dermatitis/dandruff and tinea versicolor skin infection and methyselenocysteine has been shown to reduce the growth of prostate tumors. It is also effective against asthma, chronic sinusitis, hepatitis, fibromyalgia, and arthritis. The recommended intake is between 60 to 90mcg a day. Selenium foods, Brazil nuts, shiitake mushrooms, pinto beans, chia, sunflower, sesame, and flax seeds, brown rice, cruciferous vegetables (broccoli, spinach, and cabbage) are preferred.[172a, b]

Slippery elm (*Ulmus rubra*), the inner bark, has long been used for relief of sore throat and mouth diseases. It is rich in mucilages, mainly phenolics, which work as a demulcent, a soothing film to reduce inflammation of irritated mucous membranes. The leaves may be dried and made into a powder for a tea for the digestive tract. *Caution* should be exercised as internal use may interfere with the absorption of prescription medications. It should not be used in pregnancy.[173]

***Soy** (*Glycine max*) is a legume bean containing the isoflavones, genistein and daidzein (phytoestrogens), linolenic and phytic acids, disaccharides and polysaccharides (carbohydrates), high levels of proteins with all essential amino acids, phytosterols (fats), saponins, and lots of fiber. Its antioxidant, chelation, anti-inflammatory, cholesterol, and triglyceride lowering and anticancer (lunasin) activity makes it one of the best non-animal sources of protein. Its glyceollins are antifungal and its phosphatidyl serine repairs and maintains cell membranes and brain tissue. Fermented soy foods include natto, tempeh, soybean paste, and soy sauce. The raw beans must be cooked to remove the trypsin inhibitors so that it can be digested properly. Recommended intake is between 60 to 75 mg daily. Caution should be exercised as soy allergy is common (skin and GI tract), and not used by women with a history of estrogenic tumors.[174]

Spanish needle (*Bidens pilosa*) contains over two hundred phytochemicals, some of which are polydactylene, linoleic acids, flavonoids like luteolin and butein, polyynes, terpenoids, phenolics, caffeates, and chalcone okanin, whose combined properties of antioxidant, antiseptic, and anti-inflammation activity are effective in killing cancer cells and pathogenic bacteria, improving immune system response, antifungal, hypoglycemic, hypotensive, and wound healing activity.[175]

Spearmint (*Mentha spicata*) is a common herb whose leaves and oils are have a calming effect on the stomach (indigestion, gas/flatulence, nausea), as well as in diarrhea and irritable bowel syndrome. It is used in mouth and sore throat remedies, colds with congestion, cancer, and respiratory system inflammation. It acts as an appetite stimulant, antiseptic, antioxidant, antibacterial, joint and muscle pain reliever, and antispasmodic.[176]

Stevia (S. *rebaudiana*), a sugar substitute with 150 times the sweetness of sugar, is safe and effective to use by diabetics and those with sugar sensitivities. Its leaves contain polysaccharides and glycosides, and non-sugar aglycones, which have a counteractive bitter taste. In the digestive tract, rebaudioside with high glucose becomes stevioside, with lower glucose, which is broken down into a glucose that is used by colon bacteria and therefore not absorbed, and steviol, which is excreted undigested. Stevia is much more effective and healthier than any of the warfarin-like substitutes that are ubiquitous on the market. [177]

St. John's wort (*Hypericum perforatum*) contains hypercine, hyperforine, hypericin, and high levels of flavonoids that exert their anti-depressant effect by inhibiting the uptake of MAO inhibitors, which allows more serotonin to remain in the brain tissues, that results in more elated mood. Hypericin shows active inhibition of enveloped viruses, like HSV, influenza, and HIV. It has also shown positive effects in wound healing, neuralgia and fibrositis. It is recommended for mild to moderate depression at a dose of 300mg three times daily. It works better when combined with exercise.[178]

Five-hydroxyl-L-**Tryptophan** (5-HTP) is a serotonin supplement made from the seeds of the *Griffonia simplicifolia* plant, which can boost serotonin levels in the brain, used for insomnia, depression, migraine, ADD, and obesity. It can be found in high protein foods like chicken, beef, and fish as well as in complex carbohydrates. Caution as it may have adverse effects of nausea, constipation, liver disease and aggravate asthma. Standard dose is between 50 to 400 mg a day, and is more effective at 100mg twice daily.[179]

Suma (*Hebanthe paniculata*), also known as Brazilian ginseng, is used as an energizer in counteracting fatigue related to anemia, anti-inflammation and antitumor agent. It contains nineteen amino acids, high levels of electrolytes, vitamins, and minerals, germanium to increase oxygen utilization at the cellular level, iron, saponins like pfaffosides and pfaffic acid, glycosides, and nortriterpenes. Available as an extract and in powder form, an effective dosage is 100mg per kilogram.[180]

Thyme (*Thymus vulgaris*) is an important adjunct for digestion, respiration and immune system function. It contains thymol and carvacrol, phenols, oxalic acid and diterpenes for suppressing the COX 2 expression of enzymes for reduction of inflammation, relaxation, and decongestion of respiratory muscles, astringent activity in the intestines, expectorant, antioxidant, antiseptic, and antibacterial activity. It can be taken as a tea, liquid, syrup, and oil application. There is no particular dosage.[181]

Tea tree (*Melaleuca alternifolia*) essential oil is both antibacterial and antifungal, capable of treating conventional antibiotic drug resistant infections. Its main active ingredient is terpinen-4-ol in addition to terpenes, cineoles, terpineols, pinenes, and cymene, which are active in against acne, dandruff, lice, herpes, and other skin conditions. Toxic if taken by mouth, it is available in low concentrations in soaps, skin washes and topical oils.[182]

Tobacco (*Nicotiana rustica*) is a stimulant to nerve endings, increases heart rate and alertness, releases dopamine and endorphins for pleasure, and is a painkiller for earache and toothache. It contains the addictive alkaloid nicotine, the psychoactive alkaloid harmine, and other alkaloids germacrene, anabasine, and piperidine. Caution as the risks far outweigh the benefits. It is associated with an increase in the risk of heart, lung and liver disease, several cancers, and inflammatory diseases. It is the no. 1 single most cause of preventable disease. Note that it is the toxins and carcinogens in tobacco smoke rather than nicotine that is responsible for the severity of illness and death.[183]

Trimethylglycine is an important food product found in quinoa, sugar beets, grains, and spinach. As betaine hydrochloride, it helps with digestion by producing hydrochloric acid. As glycine betaine, it neutralizes and lowers homocysteine plasma levels, which lowers risk of cardiovascular disease and stroke by protecting against excessive clotting and thrombosis.[184]

*__Turmeric__ (*Curcuma longa*) is a root plant with high levels of polyphenols and curcuminoids as its main ingredients, in addition to terpenoids, sugars, vitamin A and C, azulene, proteins, acids, and resins. Curcumin inhibits COX 2 enzymes to reduce inflammation and pain and turns on genes that keep vitamin B5 (panthothenic acid) levels stable in regulation of insulin production (diabetes). Tumerone acts on nerve cells in the brain to promote cell growth and repair (Alzheimer's). When used daily in cuisine or teas, it is very effective in preventing and treating arthritis and similar inflammatory conditions without the side effects experienced with most conventional drugs. It also offers lower cholesterol for liver and cardiovascular protection, and has anticancer, antimicrobial, and antiseptic properties. The recommended dose is one to two teaspoons of dried or powdered root daily.[185a, b, c]

Turkey rhubarb (*Rheum rhabarbarum*) contains anthraquinones, glycosides, and pectin in its stems, which have cathartic and laxative properties for constipation. In cuisine, it is used in pies and desserts and savory dishes. The leaves contain oxalic acid which is toxic to the kidneys.[186]

Turkey tail (*Trametes versicolor* or *Coriolus versicolor*) is a large mushroom with medicinal activities against cancer. As a potent immune system booster, it contains polysaccharide-K (PSK) which has been found to be effective as a treatment adjunct for gastric, lung, colorectal, breast, and lung cancers. It has been shown to reduce the risk of recurrences.[187]

Uva ursi (*Arctostaphylos uva-ursi*), also known as bearberry in North America, contains the glycodise, arbutin, which is very effective as an antimicrobial, anti-inflammatory, and mild diuretic. Used to prevent the recurrence of urinary tract and bladder infections and kidney stones, it is also effective in the treatment of the acute conditions. Though the flowers and fruit are active, it is the leaves that are infused in a tea and taken according to severity of symptoms. *Caution* should be exercised as it also contains hydroquinones, which may be toxic to the liver if taken in excess.[188]

Valerian root (*Valeriana officinalis*) contains valerianic and isovaleric acids, the alkaloids, actinidine, and chatinine, GABA, indoles, sesquiterpenes, and flavonolones, which impart sedation, anticonvulsant, antianxiety, and cramp relief actions. Effective as a smoking deterrent, it is mainly used for sleep disorders and in calming tonics for stress related conditions, like asthma, headaches, migraines, and gastric upset. The root is more potent than the leaf. A recommended effective dosage is 300 to 900mg as a tea or capsule at bedtime. It should be used for three to four consecutive nights to achieve the desired effect without the undesired side effects of conventional sleeping pills.[189]

Vanilla (*V.pianifolia*) is the second most expensive spice, after saffron. It contains vanillin, which is touted as an antioxidant, antimicrobial, antimutagenic, with specific activity against sickle cells. It is used medically to treat cancer and sickle-cell anemia.[190]

Vermicelli (*Cuscuta americana*) or love vine, contains tannins, glycosides, saponins, alkaloids, and coumarinic acid, which gives it astringent, anti-inflammatory, laxative, and liver and gall bladder protection. It is used to prevent and treat abscess, relieve constipation and liver issues.[191]

Verveine (*Verbena officinalis*) contains catechins, flavones, ursolic, salicylic, phenolic and caffeic acids, verveins, alkaloids and glycosides making it effective in hypertension and allergy control, cancer prevention and treatment, against intestinal worms and as a sedative in anxiety conditions. It may have specific neuroprotective properties against Alzheimer's dementia. Too much is toxic and should be avoided in pregnancy and in presence of cardiovascular disease.[192]

Vitamin A (beta-carotene) acts on the retina (dark adaptation), skin, tissue healing, immune system regulation, and UV radiation protection. Deficiency leads to night blindness and hardening of the nasal and respiratory surfaces. Found in yellow and green vegetables, like winter squash, broccoli, kale, spinach, carrots, sweet potatoes, eggs, liver, and dairy, the recommended daily requirement is between 10,000 to 25,000 international units (IU).

Vitamin C (ascorbic acid) acts on tissues for repair and regeneration, boosts the immune system against oxidative stress and lowers the risk of cataract formation in the eyes and C-reactive protein (toxin) in the heart. Deficiency leads to swollen gums, loose teeth, severe joint pain, and poor healing (scurvy). Found in citrus fruit and vegetables, the recommended daily requirement is between 1,000 to 1,500 mg.

Vitamin D (D3) facilitates the absorption of calcium and phosphorus for bone health, teeth development, and immune system function. It reduces the risk of developing multiple sclerosis, heart disease, and common cold and flu. It forms in the body from the absorption of sunlight in the skin. Dark skin is D deficient as pigment blocks it, while light skin absorbs faster and more readily. Deficiency leads to soft, distorted bones, referred to as rickets in children and osteomalacia in adults and fragile bones (osteoporosis) in adult, post-menopausal women. It is also found in fish oil, some mushrooms, liver, cheese, eggs, and fortified orange juice and cereals. For fair-skinned people, sun exposure should be least ten to fifteen minutes a day, and for darker complexions, thirty to forty-five minutes daily. Shut in seniors with dark complexions should take a supplement. The recommended requirement is calcitrol 600 to 800 IU.

Vitamin E (alpha-tocopherol) protects cell membranes from free radicals (oxidative stress); prevents the oxidation of LDL cholesterol; maintains skeletal, cardiac, and smooth muscle; vitamin A, K, iron, and selenium metabolism; slows cataract formation and aids in the formation of red blood cells. Deficiency leads to muscle weakness, liver disease, loss of muscle coordination, loss of tendon reflexes, and muscular dystrophy. Found in avocados, nuts, and seeds, the daily recommended requirement is between 400 IU.

Vitamin K (phylloquinone) promotes protein synthesis for platelet aggregation for blood clotting. Deficiency leads to bleeding. Found in leafy green vegetables like broccoli, spinach, and cabbage; fruit like avocado, kiwi, and grapes; and green herbs like parsley, mints, and oregano. The daily RDA is 120mcg for women and 90mcg for men.

Vitamin B1 (thiamin) regulates glucose metabolism and nerve transmission. Deficiency leads to fatigue, irritability, loss of appetite, loss of muscle function and numbness especially in the legs, mental confusion, and involuntary eye movements (beri beri). Found in wheat bran, eggs, nuts, red meat, and cereals, the recommended daily allowance (RDA) is 1.2mg.

Vitamin B2 (riboflavin) is associated with energy, vision, and skin health. Deficiency leads to cheilosis characterized by fissures at the corners of the mouth and severely chapped lips. Found in dairy, liver, vegetables, fruit, cereals, and yeast, the daily allowance (RDA) ranges from 0.3 to 0.6 in infants and children, to 1.0 mg in adults.

Vitamin B3 (niacin) is involved in cholesterol metabolism. Deficiency leads to pellagra, extreme redness, flaking and loss of skin epithelium, dermatitis, and mental confusion. Found in turkey, chicken, tuna, and crimini mushrooms, the RDA is 14 to 18 mg.

Vitamin B4 (adenine) is a coenzyme active in basic DNA and RNA metabolism for cell growth. Found in readily available whole grains, herbs, spices, raw honey, fresh fruit, and vegetables, a deficiency would manifest as growth retardation, blood and skin disease, constipation, persistent nausea and vomiting, hypoglycemia, and muscle weakness.

Vitamin B5 (panthothenic acid) coenzyme CoA is associated with proper adrenal gland function. With high levels in yeast and molds, a deficiency would involve severe fatigue, insomnia, depression, irritability, "burning feet," and frequent urinary tract infections. The RDA for adults is 5mg, in pregnancy, 6mg, and 7mg if breastfeeding.

Vitamin B6 (pyridoxine) is an antidepressant involves with tryptophan to serotonin metabolism in the brain. Deficiency results in peripheral neuropathy, seizures in infants that are unresponsive to anticonvulsant drugs. Found in meat, poultry, organ meats, enriched cereals, soy, lentils, fruit, and vegetables, the RDA of 1.3 mg for the average adult can readily be ingested from food. The maximum daily intake for pregnant and breast feeding women is upward to 100mg.

Vitamin B12 (cobalamin) is required for DNA synthesis, red blood cell development, myelination of nerves, and the production of neurotransmitters. Deficiency leads to megaloblastic anemia (abnormal size and reduced amounts of red blood cells). Found in turkey, sardines, tuna, seaweed, fruit and vegetables, the RDA is between 6 to 10 mcg.§§§[193]

Vitex (*V. agnus-castus*) contains flavonoids, alkaloids, diterpenes, and steroidal hormone precursors, which act on the pituitary gland to suppress sexual desires, hence the "chaste tree" moniker. Its dopaminergic action induces changes in prolactin secretion, which reduces symptoms of dysmenorrhea in premenstrual syndrome. Also used to treat abnormal uterine bleeding disorders, mastalgia (breast pain), and mastodynia (breast tenderness), the berries are more effective than the leaves. Caution: should not be used during pregnancy.[194]

*****Water** constitutes 75 percent of the human brain, 92 percent of blood plasma, 75 percent of muscles, and 22 percent of bones. It transports nutrients and oxygen to and from the tissues, converts food to energy, regulates body temperature, and removes waste and (lack of) is associated with approximately 70 percent of disease processes.

§§§[193] Codex Guidelines for vitamin and mineral food supplements. Codex Alimentarius Commission/United Nations. 2007.

Adequate hydration prevents and cures almost all disorders of the body and mind, like headaches, hunger, throat diseases, gut issues, arthritis, bacterial and viral infections, and heart and kidney diseases. Physical water therapy (swimming) relieves pain and muscle imbalances, reduces stress on joints, and builds muscle strength; seawater therapy offers iodine to boost thyroid activity, and increased buoyancy for exercise, and spa therapy offers relaxation for body and mind.[195a, b]

Watercress (*Nasturtium officinale*) is a vegetable of the Brassicaceae family (like broccoli and kale), known for its anticancer activity (breast, lung, and prostate) by suppression of new blood vessel formation (angiogenesis) and antioxidant action. As a stimulant with diuretic properties, it has digestive and expectorant properties as well. Containing high levels of isothiocyanates, vitamins, and minerals, essential nutrients (carbohydrates, protein, and fats), plus high levels of iron, folic acid, calcium and iodine, it also has antibacterial, anti-parasitic and anti-inflammation properties.[196]

Wheatgrass (*Thinopyrum intermedium*) contains high levels of chlorophyll, oligosaccharides, polysaccharides, vitamins, and minerals that stimulate the thyroid to boost and regulate metabolism, the immune system, alkalinizes all body systems, bind heavy metals for detoxification, and promotes healing both internally and externally. Best used fresh in salads or juiced, the general health benefits include liver protection, diabetic blood sugar regulation, thyroid regulation, digestive aid, and relief of urinary tract inflammation and infections. For prevention and regulation, initial intake of juice should not be more than one ounce a day for two to three weeks, then build up to two ounces for several weeks. Four ounces for disease control should be the limit.[197]

Whole grains are infinitely healthier than refined grains. Bran, endosperm, germ, amaranth, barley, buckwheat, corn, millet, oats (oatmeal), quinoa, brown rice , pasta, rye, sorghum (milo), teff, tritacle, wheat (spelt, emmer, farro, einkorn, famut, durkum, bulgur) are all healthful when ingested fresh and unprocessed. The high fiber content, vitamins (thiamin, riboflavin, niacin, and folate), minerals (iron, magnesium, and selenium) are active in weight management, skin health, reduced risk of heart disease, diabetic sugar control, and constipation prevention. At least three servings (45gm) a day is considered to be healthy. Caution: avoid foods made from corn, as it is now the equivalent of genetically modified organisms (GMO) in USA. On the other hand, be aware that quinoa is a gluten-free high protein fiber and is a much better choice.[198]

Wild yam root (*Dioscorea villosa*) has been used to treat menopausal symptoms of hot flashes and night sweats without scientific based evidence. The root contains diosgenin, a steroidal saponin, which has been shown to reduce adrenal gland mass (swelling), which may be the pathway to reduction in symptoms. There does not appear to be any effect on estrogenic or progesterone hormones. It also contains alkaloids, tannins, phytosterols, and starch.[199]

Willow (*Salix alba*) is the prototype for common aspirin used as a painkiller and anti-inflammation agent particularly effective in the relief of headaches, fever, joint, and low back pain. Containing salicin from the bark, which is metabolized to the active salicylic acid in the body, positive effects may be offset by side effects of gut lining irritation, blood thinning effects, and occasional allergic reactions. The synthetic acetylsalicylic acid causes less digestive upset.[200]

Wintergreen (*Gaultheria procumbens*) contains the aromatic compound, methyl salicylate, and essential oils, used for relief of upper respiratory conditions like sore throat, congestion, headache, fever, and aches. Found in mints, gums, candies, toothpaste, mouthwash, and teas, it is effective in clearing nasal passages in common colds. Caution as excess use of extracts with high levels of oil of wintergreen may be toxic especially in children.[201]

Witch hazel (*Hamamelis virginiana*) is effective for relief of symptoms of hemorrhoids, varicose veins, minor bleeding, and skin irritation from insect bites and poison ivy. Containing tannins, catechins, flavonoids, essential oils, and saponins; it has astringent and antioxidant activity. Found in numerous over-the-counter preparations, it is recommended for women to reduce swelling and soothe wounds related to childbirth.[202]

Yarrow (*Achillea millifolium*) contains chamazukene, a potent anti-inflammatory, tannins, bitter elements, asparagin, sterols, coumarins, and the alkaloid, achilletin, which together are effective in the process of hemostasis, stopping bleeding especially from the nose and gastrointestinal tract (hemorrhoids). Also with diaphoretic (for fevers) and digestive activity (promotes bile flow), yarrow can be used as a vegetable, cooked or raw.[203]

Yellow dock (*Rumex crispus*) contains toxic oxalic acid and must be boiled to remove it. Its anthroquinone glycosides, vitamins, and iron and potassium-rich proteins give it a strong astringent, antioxidant, and purgative action. It can be used to detoxify the liver, treat anemia, reduce diarrhea, heal skin eruptions, and eaten as a vegetable. *Caution* as excess use can irritate the urinary tract and form stones due to traces of oxalates remaining after boiling.[204]

Yerba maté (*Ilex paraguarensis*) contains high levels of xanthine alkaloids, decaffeolyquininc, and chlorogenic acids, caffeine, polyphenols, saponins, terpenes, vitamins C and A, and 15 amino acids. It exhibits strong antioxidant activity , elevates cellular levels of ADP, ATP, and AMO for energy boosts, suppresses adipose tissue formation for weight management, lowers LDL cholesterol, and increases nutrients to the heart to reduce the risk of cardiovascular disease, improves mood, cognition, and sleep quality, and improves digestion. The recommended use is up to three cups a day, but caution should be exercised as frequent and prolonged use may lead to mouth, throat or esophageal cancers. (205)

Yohimbe (*Pausinystalia yohimbe*) bark contains the indole alkaloid, yohimbine, which has been used traditionally as an aphrodisiac, despite lack of scientific evidence. It mechanism of action as an energizer and mild vasodilator of peripheral blood vessels, is seen in its side effects noted as increased systolic blood pressure and increased anxiety due to central nervous system stimulation.[206]

*Zinc as a prime elemental mineral is required in children to avoid growth retardation, delayed sexual maturation, infection susceptibility (colds and flu), and intractable diarrhea. Needed for the proper function of over one hundred specific enzymes, it is second only to iron as the most abundant metal in organisms. With the highest concentrations being in the prostate gland, eye, brain, muscle, kidneys and liver, it regulates apoptosis (programmed cell death) and plays a role in learning from normal brain function. Recommended dosage is 7.5 mg for colds and wound healing, 8mg a day for women, and 11mg a day for men. Found in high concentrations in oysters, lobster, beef, lamb, beans, nuts, and seeds. *Caution* should be exercised as consumption of excess zinc can lead to ataxia, lethargy, and copper deficiency. Supplementation should only be used when there is deficiency or in cases of major surgery, trauma or severe burns requiring assisted healing.[207a, b]

*These natural products have physiological actions that are especially important to natural health and disease prevention.

Common Side Effects of Natural Products

Blood Thinners: Some natural products can have additive effects on blood thinners like warfarin, heparin, coumadin, and aspirin and should be discontinued especially before undergoing surgery. An adverse effect can lead to excessive bleeding, hematoma, hematemesis, melena, thrombosis, subarachnoid hemorrhage, and subdural hematoma. Feverfew, dong quai , garlic, panax ginseng, ginkgo biloba, ginger, green tea, goji berry, chamomile, boswellia, sage, and St. John's wort are natural blood thinners to be avoided if you are taking conventional drugs and at least discussed with your physician.

Herb-Drug Interactions: Stimulants like bitter orange, guarana, kola nut, and yerba maté should not be taken with coffee as the caffeine content will be greatly magnified.

Natural antihypertensives like hibiscus, juana la blanca, and ginger should not be taken with aspirin, excedrin, pseudoephedrine, or digoxin, as the combination may lead to anxiety, insomnia, sudden fall in blood pressure, and tachycardia.

Natural immune enhancers like echinacea and astragalus may counteract the effect of corticosteroids.

Antidepressants like St. John's wort reduce the effectiveness of birth control pills and phenobarbitol.

References for Chapter 3 (NHDP)

1. Burning through the pain: treatments for diabetic neuropathy.

   a. Javed S, et al. Diabetes Obes Metab. 2015 (alpha lipoic acid)

2. A short review: Antiviral activity of aloe-emodin against influenza A virus via galactin-3-up regulation. Amar Surjushe. Et al. Indian J Dermatol. L808:3(4):163–166

3. Evolutionary history and leaf succulence as explanations for medicinal use in aloes and the global popularity of *Aloe vera*. Grace OM, et al. вcеol Biol. 2015

4. A critical review of the therapeutic potential of dibenzyl trisulphide isolated from *Petiveria alliacea* L. (guinea hen weed, anamú). Williams LA, et al, West Indian Medical J. 2007 Jan;56(1):17–21

5. *Pimpinella anisum* in the treatment of functional dyspepsia: A double-blind, randomized clinical trial. Ghoshegir SA, et al. J Res Med Sci. 2015

6. Apple cider vinegar modulates serum lipid profile, erythrocyte, kidney, and liver membrane oxidative stress in ovariectomized mice fed high cholesterol. Naziroglu M, et al. J Membr Biol. 2014

7. Effects of antioxidant compounds of AREDS vitamins and zinc ions on endothelial cell activation: implications for macular degeneration. Zeng S, et al. Invest Ophthalmol Vis Sci. 2012

8. L-Arginine and vascular diseases: lights and pitfalls! Calabro RS, et al. Acta Biomed. 2014 Dec 17; 85(3): 222–8

9. Effectiveness and Safety of *Arnica montana* in post-surgical setting: Pain and inflammation. Iannitti T, et al. Am J Ther. 2014 Sept 17

10. Dried leaf Artemesia annua: a practical malaria therapeutic for developing countries? Weathers PJ, et al. World J Pharmacol. 2014

11. Polyphenols from artichoke heads (*Cynara cardunculus Sub sp scolymus Hayek*): in vitro bio-accessibility, intestinal uptake and bioavailability. D'Antuono I, et al. Food Funct. 2015

12. Subchronic (13 week) oral toxicity study in rats with fungal chitin-glucan from *Aspergillus niger*. Jonfer D, et al. Food Chem Toxicol. 2010 Oct; 48(10):2695-701

13. Standardized extract of *Withania somnifera* (Ashwagandha) markedly offsets rotenone-induced biomotor deficits, oxidative impairments and neuro-toxicity in Drosophila melanogaster. Manjunath MJ, et alJ Food Sci Technol. 2015 Apr; 532(4): 1971–81

14. Specific Medicinal Plant Polysaccharides effectively enhance the potency of a DC-based vaccine against mouse mammary tumor metastasis. Chang WT, et al. PLos One.2015. Mar 31; 10(3)

15. Management of osteoarthritis with avocado/ soybean unsaponifiables. Christiansen BA, et al. Cartilage. 2015 (a)

    a. Effect of a moderate fat diet with and without avocados on lipoprotein particle number, size and subclasses in overweight and obese adults: a randomized, controlled trial. Wang L, et al. J Am Heart Assoc. 2015 (b)

16. Sasa qualpaertensis leaf extract inhibits colon cancer by regulating cancer cell stemness in vitro and in vivo. Min SJ, et al. Int J Mol Sci. 2015 (a) (bamboo grass)

    a. Protective effects of Bacopa monnieri on ischemia-induced cognitive deficits in mice: The possible contribution of bacopaside I and underlying mechanism. Le XT, et al. J Ethnopharmacol. 2015 (b)

17. Synergistic antibacterial effect of honey and Herba Ocimi Basilici against bacterial pathogens. Khalid AT, et al. J Tradit Chin Med. 2013 (a) (basil)

    a. Efficacy of Ocimum sanctum for relieving stress: a preclinical study. Bathala LR, et al. J Contemp Dent Pract. 2012 (b) (basil)

18. The protective effects of bilberry and lingonberry extracts against UV light-induced retinal photoreceptor cell damage in vitro. Ogawa K, et al. J Agric Food Chem. 2013 (a)

    a. Effects of bilberry on deoxyribonucleic acid damage and oxidant-antioxidant balance in the lens, induced by ultraviolet radiation. Aly EM, et al. Malays J Med Sci. 2014 (b)

19. Black cohosh: an alternative therapy for menopause? Mahady GB, et al. Nutr Clin Care. 2002

20. Anticancer effect of black tea extract in human cancer cell lines. Konarikova K, et al. Springerplus. 2015

21. Antioxidant levels of common fruits, vegetables and juices versus protective activity against in vitro ischemia/reperfusion. Bean H, et al. Int Urol Nephrol. 2010 (blueberry)

22. Oral herbal therapies for treating osteoarthritis. Cameron M, et al. Cochrane Summaries, May 22, 2014

23. The epigenetic impact of cruciferous vegetables on cancer prevention. Royston KJ, et al. Curr Pharmacol Rep. 2015 (broccoli)

24. Spirostanol saponinsand esculin from rusci rhizome reduc the thrombin-induced hyperpermeability of endothelial cells. Barbic M, et al. Phytochemistry 2013. (butchers broom)

25. Antiallergic and anti-inflammatory effects of bakkenolide B isolated from *Petasites japonicas* leaves. Lee KP, et al. J Ethnopharmacol. 2013 (butterbur)

26. Calcium and health. Ortega Anta RM, et al. Nutr Hosp. 2015

27. Extracts of *Calendula officinalis* offer in vitro protection against H2O2 induced oxidative stress cell killing of human skin cells. Alnuqaydan AM, et al. Phytother Res. 2015

28. Medical and recreational marijuana: commentary and review of literature. Wilkinson ST, et al. Mo Med. 2013

29. Antimutagenic and antiherpetic activities of different preparations from *Uncaria tomentosa* (Cat's Claw). Caon T, et al. Food Chem Toxicol. 2014

30. Biological activities of red pepper (*Capsicum annuum*) and its pungent principle capsaicin: A review.

Srinivasan K, et al. Crit Rev Food Sci Nutr. 2015 (cayenne pepper)

31. Larvicidal, repellant, and irritatant potential of a seed-derived essential oil of Apium graveolens against dengue fever vector, Aedes aegypti L. Kumar S, et al. Front Public Health. 2014 (a)

   a. Antimicrobial and P450 inhibitory properties of common functional foods. Nguyen S, et al. J Pharm Pharm Sci. 2014 (b) (celery seed, cumin, fennel, basil, oregano, rosemary)

32. Consumption of whole grains and cereal fiber and total and cause specific mortality: prospective analysis of 367,442 individuals. Huang T, et al. BMC Med. 2015

33. A review of the bioactivity and potential health benefits of chamomile tea (*Matricaria recutita*). McKay DL, et al. Phytotherapy Research. 2006; 20(7): 519-520 (a)

   a. Study of anti-seizure effects of *Matricaria recutita* extract in mice. Heidari MR, et al. Am NY Acad Sci. 2009 (b)

34. Effects of chocolate intake on perceived stress; a controlled clinical study. Al Sunni A, et al. Int J Health Sci. 2014

35. Effect of chromium supplement on blood glucose and lipid levels in type 2 diabetes mellitus elderly patients. Rabinovitz H, et al. Int J Vitam Nutr Res. 2004

36. Dimeric Cinchona alkaloids. Boratynski PH, et al. J Mol Divers. 2015

37. Cinnamic acid exerts anti-diabetic activity by improving glucose tolerance in vivo and by stimulating insulin secretion in vitro. Hafizier RM, et al. Phytomedicine. 2015 (cinnamon)

38. Clove *(Eugenia aromatica)* and clove oil (eugenol). Natural Standard monograph. Basich E, et al. J Diet Suppl. 2008

39. Biological activity of the alkaloids of Erythroxylum coca and Erythroxylum novogranatense. Novain M, et al. J Ethnopharmacol. 1984 (a)

    a. The therapeutic value of coca in contemporary medicine. Weil, AT (mar–may 1981) J Ethnopharmacol 3 (2-3): 367–76 (b)

40. Tissue invasion and metastasis: Molecular, Biological and Clinical perspectives. Jiang WG, et al. Semin Cancer Biol. 2015 (a)

    a. A pilot study: the efficacy of virgin coconut oil as ocular rewetting agent on rabbit eyes.

Mutalib HA, et al. Evid Based Complement Alternat Med 2015. (b)

41. Effects of Coenzyme Q10 supplementation on serum lipoprotein, plasma fibrinogen, and blood pressure in patients with hyperlipidemia and myocardial infarction. Mohensi M, et al. Iran Red Crescent Med J. 2014

42. Coffee components and Cardiovascular risk: beneficial and detrimental effects. Godos J, et al. Int J Food Sci Nutr. 2014

43. NYU Langone Medical Centr. "Coleus Forskohlii." Godard M, Obesity Research, August 2005.

44. A critical scoping review of external use of comfrey (Symphytum). Frost R, et al. Complement Ther Med.2013

45. A randomized, double-blind, placebo-controlled trial to assess the bacterial anti-adhesion effect of cranberry extract beverages. Kaspar KL, et al. Food Funct 2015.

46. A comparative study of the anti-microbial, antioxidant, and cytotoxic activities of methanol extracts from fruit bodies and fermented mycelia of caterpillar medicinal mushroom Cordyceps militaris (Ascomycetes). Dong CH, et al. Int J Med Mushrooms. 2014

47. Contents of Damiana drugs. Auterhoft H, et al. Arch Pharm Ber Dtsch Pharm Ges. 1968 Jul: 301(7): 637.44

48. Effect of leaf extract of Taraxacum officinalis on CC L4 induced hepatotoxicity in rats, in vivo study. Gulfraz M, et al. J Pharm Sci. 2014 (dandelion)

49. Endocrine factors, memory and perceptual capacities and aging in Asian men. Goh VH, et al. Aging Male. 2015 (a)

    a. The DHEA-sulfate depot following P450c17 inhibition supports the case for AFR1C3 inhibition in high risk localized and advanced castration resistant prostate cancer. Tamae D, et al. Chem Biol Interact. 2014 (b)

50. Phytochemical and pharmacological studies on Radix Angelica sinensis. Chen XP, et al. Chin J Nat Med. 2013 (dong quai)

51. Immune enhancing effects of Echinacea purpura root extract by reducing regulatory T cell number and function. Kim HR, et al. at Prod Commun. 2014

52. Cholesterol feeding reduces nuclear forms of sterol regulating element binding proteins in hamster liver. Shimomura I, et al. Biochem Proc Nat'l Acad Sci USA 1997 Nov 11; 94 (23) (eggs)

53. Antiinfluenza virus effects of elderberry juice and its fractions. Kinoshita E, et al. Bioscience, Biotech, and Biochem 76(9):1633-1638. 7 Sept 2012

54. Bioactive compounds and antioxidative, antileukemic and anti-MPs activity of Eleutherococcus species cultivated in Poland. Zaluski D, et al/ Nat Prod Commun. 2012

55. The anti=obesity effect of Ephedra sinica through modulaton of gut microbiota in obese Korean women. Kim BS, et al. J Ethnopharmacol. 2014

56. Antimicrobial and Antioxidant activities and phenolic profile of Eucalyptus glabulus labilli and Corymbia ficifolia leaves. Dezsi S, et al. Molecules. 2015

57. Evening primrose oil and celecoxib inhibited pathological angiogenesis, inflammation and oxidative stress in adjuvant-induced arthritis: novel role of angiopoietin-1. E-Sayed RM, et al. Inflammopharmacology. 2014

58. Foen vul Mill: a review of its botany, phytochemistry, pharmacology, contemporary application, and toxicology. Badgujar SB. Et al/ Biomed Rs Int. 2014 (fennel)

59. Influence of a specialized Trigonella foenum graecum seed extract (Libifem) on testosterone, estradiol and sexual function in healthy menstruating women,

a randomized placebo controlled study. Rao A, et al. Phytother Res. 2015 (fenugreek)

60. Feverfew for preventing migraine. Wider B, et al. Cochrane Database Syst Rev. 2015

61. Whole grain consumption and breast cancer; a case-controlle study in women. Mourouti N, et al. J Am Coll Nutr. 2015

62. Flaxseed- a potential functional food source. Kajla P. et al. J Food Sci Technol. 2015

63. Folate status and concentrations of serum folate forms in the US population: National Health and nutrition examination survey 2011-2012 Pfeiffer CM, et al. Br J Nutr. 2015

64. Chasing cardiac physiology and pathology down the CaMF II cascade. Mattiazzi A, et al. Am J Physiol Heart Circ Physiol. 2015 (foxglove)

65. A comprehensive scientific overview of Garcinia cambrogia. Semuel RB, et al. Filoterapia. 2015

66. Antimicrobial properties of allicin from garlic. Ankri S, et al. Microbes Infect 2)2):125-9 (1999) (a)

   a. Effects of garlic oil on interleukin-6 mediated cardiac hypertrophy in hyperchlesterol-fed hamsters. Hsieh YL, et al. Chin J Physiol. 2014 (b)

b. Antibacterial activity of a new, stable, aqueous extract of allicin against methicillin resistant staphylococcus aureus. Cutler RR, et al. Br J Biomed Sci 52(3):71-74/ 2004 (c)

67. Comparative HPLC/ESI-MS and HPLC? DAD study of different populations of cultivated, wild and commercial Gentiana lutea L. Mustafa AM, et al. Food Chem. 2015

68. A comparative study of Zinziber officinale Roscoe pupl and peel: phytochemical composition and evaluation of antitumor activity. Marrelli M, et al. Nat Prod Res. 2015 (a)

    a. Is ginger beneficial for nausea and vomiting? An update of the literature. Marx N, et al. Curr Opin Support Palliat Care 2015 (b)

69. Systematic review of pharmacologic and non-pharmacologic interventions to manage cognitive alterations after chemotherapy for breast cancr. Chan RJ, et al. Eur J Cancer. 2015 (ginkgo b)

70. Ginseng: a promising neuroprotective strategy in stroke. Rastogi V, et al. Front Cell NeuroSci. 2014

71. Glucosamine and chondroitin sulfate supplementation to treat symptomatic disc degeneration: biochemical rational and case report. Van Bitterswijk WJ, et al. BMC Complement Altern Med. 2003. (a)

a. What is the current status of chondroitin sulfate and glucosamine for the treatment of knee osteoarthritis? Henrotin Y, et al. Maturitas. 2014 (b)

72. Biflorin: an o-naphthoquinone of clinical significance. Wisintainer GG, et al. An Acad Bras Cienc. 2014

73. Practical application of Antidiabetic efficacy of Lycium barbarum polysaccharide in patients with type 2 diabetes. Cai H, et al. Med Chem. 2015 (a) (gojiberry)

a. Dietary supplementation with lacto-wolfberry enhances the immune response and reduces pathogenesis to influenza infection in mice. Ren Z, et al. J Nutr, 2012 (b)

74. Hydrastine pharmacokinetics and metabolism after a single oral dose of goldenseal (Hydrastis canadiensis) to humans. Gupta K, et al. Drug Metab Dispos. 2015

75. Protective effects of Phyllanthus emblica leaf extract on sodium arsenite-mediated adverse effects in mice. Sayed S, et al. Nagoya J Med Sci. 2015 (a) (gooseberry)

a. a.Phyllanthus spp. Induces selective growth inhibition of PC-3 and MeWo human cancer cells through modulation of cell cycle and induction of apoptosis. Tang YQ, et al. PLos One. 2010 (b)

76. Pycnogenol and Centella asiatica for asymptomatic atherosclerosis progression. International Angiology. 33(1):20-26. Feb 2014 (gotu kola)

77. The effects of grapefruits (Citrus paradise) on body weight and cardiovascular risk factors: A systematic review and meta-analysis of randomized clinical trials. Onakpoya I, et al. Crit Rev Food Sci Nutr. 2015 (a)

   a. Grapefruit juice improves glucose intolerance in streptozotocin-induced diabetes by suppressing hepatic gluconeogenesis. Hayanga JA, et al. Eur J Nutr. 2015 (a)

78. Platelet reactivity in male smokers following the acute consumption of a flavonol-rich grapeseed extract. Pearson DA, et al. Clin Dev Immunol. 2005 (a)

   a. Grapeseed proanthocyanidin extract protects human lens epithelium from oxidative stress via reducing NF-kB and MAPK protein expression. Jia Z, et al. Mol Vis. 2011 (b)

79. Synergistic interactions among flavonoids and acetogenins in Graviola (Annona muricata) leaves confer protection against prostate cancer. Yang C, et al. Carcinogenesis. 2015

80. Green tea catechins and sport performance. Books & documents. Adisa A, et al. Antioxidants in Sport Nutrition. 2015 (a)

    a. The safety of green tea extract supplementation in postmenopausal women at risk for breast cancer: results of the Minnesota Green tea trial. Dostal AM, et al. Food hem Toxicol. 2015 (b)

81. Anti-malarial activity of a poly-herbal product (Nefang) during early and established Plasmodium infecton rodent models. Tarkang PA, et al. Malar J 2014

82. Resin from the mukul myrrh tree, guggul, can it be used for treating hypercholesterolemia? A Neuroprotective effects of citrus flavonoids. Hwang SL, et al. J of Agricul and Food Chem 60(4):877-85. 2012randomized, controlled study. Nohr LA, et al. Complement Ther Med. 2009

83. A review of the chemistry of the genus Crataegus. Edwards IE, et al. Phytochemitry 2012 (a)

    a. A randomized double blind placebo controlled clinical trial of a standardized extract of fresh Crataegus berries (Crataegisan) in the treatment of patients with congestive heart failure NYHAII. Degenring FH, et al. Phytomedicine 2003 (b)

84. Neuroprotective effects of citrus flavonoids. Hwang SL, et al. J of Agricul and Food Chem 60(4):877-85 2012 (a)

   a. Neuropharmacologica properties and pharmacokinetics if the citrus flavonoids hesperidin and hesperetin. A mini review. Roohbakhsh A, et al. Life Sciences 113 (1-2): 1-6. 2014 (b)

85. Effect of sour tea (H. sabdariffa L.) on arterial hypertension: a systematic review and meta- analysis of randomized controlled trials. Serban G, et al. J Hypertens 2015 (a)

   a. The triterpenoids of Hibiscus syriacus induce apoptosis and inhibit cell migration in breast cancer cells. Hsu RJ, et al. BMC Complement Altern Med. 2015

86. Methyglyoxal: (active agent of Manuka honey) in vitro activity against bacterial biofilms. Internat'l Forum of Allergy & Rhinology 1(5)"348-350. 2011 (a)

   a. Honey as a topical treatment for wounds. Cochrane database. Jull AB, et al. Oct 8, 2008 (b)

87. (Chinese Herbal Medicine Formulas + Strategies (2nd Ed.) Eastland Press p.44. Bensky D. et al

a. Honeysuckle-encoded atypical microRNA 2911 directly targets influenza A virus. Zhou Z, et al. Cell Res. 2015 (a)

b. Anti-proliferative activity of hydnocarpin, a natural lignin, is associated with the suppression of Wnt/B-catenin signaling pathway in colon cancer cells. Lee MA, et al. Bioorg Med Chem Lett. 2013 (b)

88. The effect of Hop (Humulus lupulus) on early menopausal symptoms and hot flashes: A randomized placebo-controlled rial. Aghamiri V, et al. Complement Ther Clin Pract. 2015 (a)

a. Anti-proliferative activity of hop-derived prenylflavonoids against human cancer cell lines.

b. Busch C, et al. Wien Med Wochensch. 2015 (b)

89. Rutosides for prevention of post-thrombotic syndrome. Morling JR, et al. Cochrane Database Syst Rev . 2013 (a)

a. Non=pharmacentical measures for prevention of post-thrombotic syndrome. Kolbach DN, et al. Cochrane Database. 2014 (b)

90. [From nasal irrigation to horseradish poultice: prescriptions for nasal congestion] Meyer F, et al. Fortscher Med. 2007 (article in German)

91. Antioxidative and antiproliferative activities of different horsetail (Equisetum arvense) extracts. Cetojevic-Simin DD, et al. J Med Food, 2010 (a)

    a. Horsetail: Univ of Md Med Center. Ehrlich SD, Complimentary and Alternative Medicine Guide, 5 March 2011. (b)

92. Assessment of the adrenergic beta-blocking activity of Inula racemose. Tripathi YB, et al. J Ethnopharmacol. 1988

93. Effect of oral Pilocarpine in treating severe Dry Eye in patients with Sjogren Syndrome. Kawakitu T, et al. Asia Pac J Ophthalmol (Phila). 2015 (jaborandi)

94. UPLC-DAD/Q-TOF-MF Based ingredients iden-tification and vasorelaxant effect of ethanol extract of jasmine flower. Yin Y, et al. Evid Based Complement Altern Med. 2014

95. The healing power of rainforest plants. Taylor L, 2005 (jatoba)

96. Plantas medicinales de Puerto Rico, Melendez EN, 1943 (juana la blanca)

97. Essential oil from berries of Lebanese Juniperus excels M. Bieb displays similar antibacterial activ-

ity of Chlorhexidrine but higher cyto-compatibility with human oral primary cells. Azzimontii B, et al. Molecules. 2015 (juniper berry)

98. Therapeutic potential of kava in the treatment of anxiety disorders. Singh YN, et al. CNS drugs. 2002

99. Evaluation of antioxidant activity of Picrorrhiza kurroa (leaves) extracts. Kant K, et al. Indian J Pharm sci. 2013 (kutaki)

100. Association of lecithin-cholesterol acyltransferase activity measured as a serum cholesterol esterification rate and low-density lipoprotein heterogeneity with cardiovascular risk: a cross-sectional study. Tani S, et al. Heart Vessels. 2015

101. Dietary patterns after prostate cancer diagnosis in relation to disease-specific and total mortality. Yang M, et al. Cancer Prev Res (Phila). 2015

102. Effect on blood pressure of daily lemon ingestion and walking. Kato Y, et al. J Nutr Metab. 2014

103. Melissa officinalis extract inhibits attachment of herpes simplex virus in vitro. Astani A, et al. Chemotherapy. 2012 (a)Melissa officinalis extract in the treatment of patients with mild to moderate Alzheimer's disease: a double blind, randomized, placebo controlled trial. Akhondzadeh S, et al. J Neurol NeuroSurg Psychiatry. 2003 (b)

104. The in vitro antimicrobial activity of Cymbopogon essential oil (lemon grass) and its interaction with silver ions. Ahmad A, et al. Phytomedicine. 2015 (a) i.Ethnopharmacology, phytochemistry and biological activities of Cymbopogon cirates (DC) Stapf extracts. Ekpenyong CE, et al. Chin J Nat Med. 2015

105. A drug over the millennia: pharmacognosy, chemistry and pharmacology of licorice. Shibata S, et al. J of Pharmaceutical Society of Japan 2000, 120 (10): 849-862

106. Mechanisms underlying the antinociceptive, antiedematogenic, and anti inflammatory activity of the main flavonoid from Kalanchoe pinnata. Ferreira RT, et al. Evid Based Complement Altern Med 2014

107. Different effects of lobeline on neuronal and muscle nicotinic receptors. Kaniakova M, et al. Eur J Pharmacol 2014

108. Carotenoid consumption is related to lower lipid oxidation and DNA damage in middle-aged men. Cocate PG, et al. Br J Nutr. 2015 (a)

     a.   Sustained supplementation and monitored response with differing carotenoid formulations in early age-related macular degeneration. Akuffo KO, et al. Eye (Lond). 2015 (b)

109. Lycopene inhibits disease progression in patients with benign prostate hyperplasia. Schwarz S, et al. J Nutr. 2008 (a)

  a. Carotenoid profile of tomato sauces: effect of cooking time and contents of extra virgin olive oil. Vallverdu-Queralt A, et al. Int J Mol Sci. 2015

110. A double-blind placebo controlled trial of maca root as treatment for antidepressant-induced sexual dysfunction in women. Dording CM, et al. Evid Based Complement Alternat Med. 2015 (a)

  a. Lepidium meyenii (Maca) enhances the serum levels of luteinizing hormone in female rats. Uchiyama F, et al. J Ethnopharmacol. 2014 (b)

111. Free radical scavenging activity, metal chelation and antioxidant power of some of the Indian spices. Yadav AS, et al. Biofactors. 2007 (a)

  a. Effects of mace and nutmeg on human cytochrome p450 3A4 and 2C9 activity. Kimura Y, et al. Biol Pharm Bull. 2010 (b)

112. The relationship between dietary magnesium intake, stroke and its major risk factors, blood pressure and cholesterol, in the EPIC-Norfolk cohort. Bain K, et al. Int J Cardiol. 2015

113. Differential anti-diabetic effects and mechanism of action of charantin-rich extract of Taiwanese Mormordica charantia between type 1amd type 2 diabetic mice. Wang HY, et al. Food Chem Toxicol 2014

114. Phytochemicals from Mangifera pajang kosterm and their biological activities. Ahmad S, et al. BMC Complement Altern Med, 2015 (mango)

115. LC-MS-based metabolite profiling of methanolic extract from the medicinal and aromatic species Mentha pulegium and Origanum majorana, Taamalli A, et al. Phytochem Anal. 2015

116. Evaluation of the antibacterial activity of the Althaca officinalis leaf extract and its wound healing potency in the rat model of excision wound creation. Rezaei M, et al. Avicenna J Phytomed. 2015 (marshmallow)

117. Chronic melatonin treatment prevents memory impairment induced by chronic sleep deprivation. Alzoubi KH, et al. Mol Neurobiol. 2015 (a)

   a.   Melatonin decreases cell proliferation, impairs myogenic differentiation and triggers apoptotic cell death in rhabdomyosarcoma cell lines. Codenotti S, et al. Oncol Rep. 2015 (b)

118. Effect of Liverubin on hepatic biochemical profile in patients of alcoholic liver disease: a retrospective study. Nanda V, et al. Minerva Med. 2014 (a)

a.　Effects and tolerance of silymarin (milk thistle) in chronic hepatitis C virus infection patients: a meta-analysis of randomized controlled trials. Yang Z, et al. Biomed Res Int. 2014 (b)

119. 2'-Hydroxy flavanone derivatives as inhibitors of pro-inflammatory mediators: Patel NK, et al. Bio Org Med Chem Lett. 2015 (Mimosa pudica)

120. Cultivation, genetic, ethnopharmacology, phyto-chemistry and pharmacology of Moringa oleifera leaves: An overview. Leone A, et al. Int J Mol Sci. 2015 (a)

a.　Health benefits of Moringa oleifera. Abdull Razis AF, et al. Asian Pac J Cancer Prev. 2014 (b)

121. Methysulfonyl methane modulates apoptosis of LPS/IFN-y-activated RAW 264.7 macrophage-like cells by targeting p53, Bax, Bel-2, cytochrome c and PARP proteins. Karabay AZ, et al. Immunopharmacol Immunotoxicol. 2014 (MSM)

122. Antiviral effect and mode of action of methanolic extract of Verbascum thapsis on pseudo rabies virus (strain RC/79) Escobar FM, et al. Nat Prod Res. 2012 (mullein)

123. Prunus mume extract ameliorates exercise-induced fatigue in trained rats. Soyoung K, et al. J of Med Food. 2008 (a)

a.   Inhibition of Heliobactor pylori motility by Syringaresinol Prom unripe Japanese apricot. Miyazawa M, et al. Bio & Pharmacol Bull. 2006 (b)

124. Administration of a polysaccharide from Grifola frondosa stimulates immune function of normal mice. Kodama N, et al. J of Med Food 7(2), 2004 (a) (maitake mushroom)

a.   Consuming Lentinula edodes (Shiitake) mushrooms daily improves human immunity: a randomized dietary intervention in healthy young adults. Dai X, et al. J Am Coll Nutr. 2015 (b)

b.   Anti-inflammatory effects of Ganoderma lucidum triterpoid in human Crohn's disease associated with down regulation of NF-kB signaling. Liu C, et al. Inflamm Bowel Dis. 2015 (c) (reischii)

125. Analgesic effects of myrrh. Dolara P, et al. Nature. 1996 (a)

a.   Hypocholesterolemic effect of some plants and their blend as studied in albino rats. Amoudi NS, et al. Int;l J of Food Safety, Nutr & Pub Health/ 2009 (b)

126. Thrombolytic effects in vivo of nattokinase in a carrageeran-induced rat model of thrombosis. Xu J, et al. Acta Haematol. 2014 (natto)

127. Organic neem compounds inhibit soft-rot fungal growth and improve the strength of anthracite bricks bound with collagen and lignin for use in iron foundry cupolas. Kelsey DJ, et al. J Appl Microbiol, 2015

128. Mechanism of action of stinging nettles. Cummings AJ, et al. Wilderness Environ Med. 2011

129. Noni (Morinda citrifolia) fruit extract improve colon microflora and exert anti inflammatory activities in Caco-2 cells. Huang HL, et al. J Med Food. 2015

130. Antimicrobial screening of different extract of Anacardium occidentale leaves. Akash P, et al. Int'l J Chem Tech Res 2009 (a)

    a. Phenolics of green husk in mature walnut fruit. Cosmulescu S, et al. Not Bot Hort Agrobot Cluj, 2010 (b)

    b. Effect of pistachio nut consumption in endothelial function and arterial stiffness. Kasiwal RR, et al. Nutrition. 2015 (c)

131. Can dietary oats promote health? Welch RW, Br J Biomed Sci 1994 (a)

a.   Wheat bran: its composition and benefits to health, a European perspective. Stevenson L, et al. Int J Food Sci Nutr. 2012 (b)

132. Mediterranean dietary pattern for the primary prevention of cardiovascular disease. Rees K, et al. Cochrane database Syst Rev. 2013 Aug 12; 8

133. Omega-3 fatty acids _ a review of existing and innovative delivery methods. Lane KE, et al. Crit Rev Food Sci Nutr. 2015 (a)

a.   Omega-3 polyunsaturated fatty acid supplementation and cognition: A systematic review and meta-analysis. Cooper RE, et al. J Psychopharmacol. 2015 (b)

134. Evaluation of quercetin as a countermeasure to exercise induced physiological stress. Konrad M, et al. Antioxidants in Sport Nutritin 2015 (a)

a.   Onion: nature protection against physiological threats. Suleria HA, et al. Crrt Rev Food Sci Nutr. 2015 (b)

135. Composition, antimicrobial, antioxidant, and antiproliferative activity of Origanum diotamnus essential oil. Mitropoulou G, et al. Microb Ecol Health Dis. 2015 (oregano)

136. Evaluation of benefits and risks related to seafood consumption. Sioen I, et al. Vesh K, Acad Geneeskd Belg 2007 (oysters)

137. Antioxidant and antibacterial activity of Rhoeo spathacea (Swartz) Stearn leaves. Tan JB, et al. J Food Sci Technol. 2015

138. Antiinflammatory and antioxidant properties of unripe papaya exract in an excision wound model. Nafiu AB, et al. Pharm Biol. 2015

139. Pharmacological importance of an ethnobotanical plant: Capsicum annuum. Khan FA, et al. Nat Prod Res. 2014 (paprika)

140. Petroselinum crispum has antioxidant properties, protects against DNA damage and inhibits proliferation and migration of cancer cells. Tang EL, et al. J Sci Food Agric 2015

141. Passiflora incarnate: ethnopharmacology, clinical application, safety and evaluation of clinical trials. Miroddi M, et al. J Ethnopharmacol. 2013

142. Downregulation of Sp 1 is involved in Beta-lapachone-induced cell cycle arrest and apoptosis in oral squamous cell carcinoma. Jeon YJ, et al. Int J Oncol. 2015

143. Plants used for treatment of dysentery and diarrhea by the Bhoxa community of district

Dehradun, Uttarakhand, India. Gairola S, et al. J Ethnopharmacol. 2013

144. Peppermint antioxidants revisited. Riachi LG, et al. Food Chem 2015

145. Interactions of the CAtharanthus (vinca) alkaloids with tubules and microtubules. Himes RH, et al. Pharmacol Ther. 1991 (a)

  a. Inhibitors of microtubule polymerization-new natural compounds as potential anti-cancer drugs. Rogalska A, et al. Postepy Hg Med Dosw. 2015

146. Isolation and structural elucidation of cytotoxic compounds from the root bark of Diospyros queruna endemic to Madagascar. Ruphin FP, et al. Asian Pac J Trop Biomed. 2014

  a. (persimmon)

147. Pharmacokinetic, bioavailability, metabolism and plasma protein binding evaluation of NADPH-oxidase inhibitor apocynin using LC-MS/MS. Chandasona H, et al. J Chromatogr B Analyt Technol Biomed Life Sci. 2015 (a) (picrorrhiza)

  a. Cardioprotective effect of root extract of Picrorrhiza kurroa against isoproterenol-induced cardiotoxicity in rats. NAndave M, et al. Indian J Exp Biol. 2013 (b)

148. Bromelain: a natural proteolytic for intra-abdominal adhesions prevention. Sahbaz A, et al. Int J Surg . 2015 (a)

    a.   Bromelain Monograph: Altern Med Rev. 2010 (b)

149. In vitro effects of plantago major extract on urolithiasis. Aziz SA, et al. Malays J Med Sci. 2005 (plantain)

150. The effect of pomegranate fruit extract on testosterone-induced BPH in rats. Aman AE, et al. Prostate. 2015 (a)

    a.   Punica granatum w. dente di Cavallo seed ethanolic extract: antioxidant and antiproliferative activities. Lucci P, et al. Food Chem. 2015 (b)

    b.   Potential anti-inflammatory effects of the hydrophilic fraction of pomegranate (Punica granatum) seed oil on breast cancer cell lines. Costantini S, et al. Molecules. 2014 ©

151. Interactions between innate immunity, microbiota, and probiotics. Giorgetti G, et al. J Immunol Res. 2015 (a)

    a.   Clinical usefulness of probiotics against chronic inflammatory bowel diseases. Mach T, et al. J Physiol and Pharmacol. 2006 (b)

b.   Probiotics as functional food in the treatment of diarrhea. Yan F, et al. Curr Opin Clin Nutr and Metab Care. 2006 (c)

152. Randomized clinical trial: dried prunes vs psyllium for constipation. Attaluri A, et al. Aliment Pharmacol Ther. 2011

153. Effect of psyllium on glucose and serum lipid responses in men with type 2 diabetes and hypercholesterolemia. Anderson JW, et al. Am J Clin Nutr. 1999

154. Homoisoflavonoids from the medicinal plant Portulaca oleracea. Yan J, et al. Phytochemistry. 2012 (a) (purslane)

a.   The effect of purslane seeds on glycemic status and lipid profiles of persons with type 2 diabetes: A randomized controlled cross-over clinical trial. Esmaillzadeh A, et al. J Res Med Sci. 2015 (b)

155. Quercetin prevents adipogenesis by regulation of transcriptional factors and lipases of OP9 cells. Seo YS, et al. Int J Mol Med . 2015 (a)

a.   Quercetin and related polyphenols: new insights and implications for their bioactivity and bioavailability. Kawabata K, et al. Food Funct. 2015

156. Nutritional quality of the protein in Quinoa (Chenopodium quino) seeds. Ruales J, et al. Plant Foods Hum Nutr. 1992

157. Raspberry leaf in pregnancy: its safety and efficacy in labor. Simpson M, et al. J of Midwifery and Womens health. 2001

158. Red clover extract for alleviating hot flushes in post-menopausal women: a meta-analysis. Gartoulla P, et al. Maturitas 2014 (a)

    a. Effects of extracts from Trifolium medium and Trifolium pretense ondevelopment of estrogen-deficiency-induced osteoporosis in rats. Cegiela U, et al. Evid Based Compl Altern Med. 2012. (b)

159. Resveratrol reverses morphine-induced neuroin-flammation in morphine-tolerant rats by reversal HDAC1 expression. Tsai RY, et al. J Formos Med Assoc. 2015

160. Traditional Chinese lipid-lowering agent red yeast rice results in significant LDL reduction but safety is uncertain_A systematic reviewand meta-analysis. Gerards MC, et al. Atherosclerosis. 2015

161. Pharmacokinetics of active constituents of Rhodiola rosea L. special extract SHR-5. In:Comprehensive Bioactive Natural Products Vol.2:Efficacy, Safety

& Clinical Evaluation (Part I). Panossian A, et al. Studium Press LLC, USA, 2010.

162. Pharmacology of rosemary (Rosmarinus off.) and its therapeutic potentials. Al-Sereiti MR, et al. Indian J Exp Biol. 1999 (a)

   a. Brainfood for Alzheimer-free Aging: focus on herbal medicines. Hügel HM. Adv Exp Med Biol. 2015 (b)

   b. Rosmarinus officinalis leaf extract improves memory impairment and affects acetylcholinesterase and butyrylcholinesterase activities in rat brain. Ozarowski M, et al. Filoterapia. 2013 (c)

163. The ocular hypotensive effect of saffron extract in primary open angle glaucoma: a pilot study. Jabbarpoor Bonyadi MH, et al. BMC Complement Altern Med. 2014

164. Effect of Carthamus tinctorius (Safflower) on fasting blood glucose and insulin levels in alloxan induced diabetic rabbits. Qazi N, et al. Pak J Pharm Sci. 2014

165. Protective properties of Salvia lavandulifolia essential oil against oxidative stress-induced neuronal injury. Porres-Martinez M, et al. Food Chem Toxicol. 2015 (a)

a. Teotihuacanin, a diterpene with an unusual spiro-10/6 system from salvia amarissima with potent modulatory activity of multidrug resistance in cancer cells. Bautista E, et al. Org Lett. 2015 (b)

166. S-adenosylmethionine (SAMe) versus calexcoxib for the treatment of osteoarthritis symptoms: a double blind cross-over trial. Najm WI, et al. BMC Musculoskelet Discord. 2004 (a)

a. Is S-adenosylmethionine (SAMe) for depression only effective in males? A re-analysis of data from a randomized clinical trial. Sarris J, et al. Pharmacopsych 2015 (b)

167. Antioxidant and cytotoxic activity of stems of Smilax zeylanica in vitro. Uddin MN, et al. J Basic Clin Physiol Pharmacol. 2015 (sarsaparilla)

168. Safrole-2', 3'-oxide induces cytotoxic and genetoxic effects in HepG2 cells and in mice. Chiang SY, et al. Mutat Res. 2011 (sassafras)

169. Anti-inflammation properties of lipidosterolic extract of Serenoa repens in a mouse model of prostate hyperplasia. Bernichtein S, et al. Prostate. 2015 (Saw palmetto)

170. Schizandrin C ameliorates learning and memory deficits by AB1-4Z-induced oxidative stress and neurotoxicity in mice. Mao X, et al. Phytother Res.

2015 (b) The antioxidative effect and ingredients of oil extracted from Schizandra chinensis. Ryu IH, (Korea)

171. Kelp use in patients with thyroid cancer. Rosen JE, et al. Endocrine. 2014

   a.   Synergy between sulforaphane and selenium in protection against oxidative damage in colonic CCD 841 cells. Wang Y, et al. Nutr Res. 2015 (b) Evidence that selenium binding protein 1 is a tumor suppressor in prostate cancer. Ansong E, et al. PLos One. 2015

172. Characterization of phenolics in Flor-Essence_ a compound herbal product and its contributing herbs. Saleem A, et al. Phytochem Anal. 2009 (Slippery elm)

173. Functional components and medicinal properties of food: a review. Abuajah CI, et al. J Food Sci Technol. 2015 (soy)

174. Investigation of the extracts from Bidens pilosa radiate Sch Bip for antioxidant activities and cytotoxicity against human tumor cells. Wu J, et al. J Nat Med. 2013 (Spanish needle)

175. High rosmarinic acid-spearmint tea in the management of Knee osteoarthritis symptoms. Connelly AE, et al. J Med Food. 2014

176. Isolation and characterization of inulin with a high degree of polymerization from roots of stevia rebaudiana. Lopes SM, et al. Carbohydr Res. 2015

177. Hypericins: biotechnological production from cell and organ cultures. Murthy HM, et al. Appl Microbiol Biotechnol. 2014

178. Etiological classification of depression based on the enzymes of tryptophan metabolism. Fukuda K, BMC Psychiatry. 2014

179. Effects of Pfaffia paniculata (Brazilian ginseng) extract on macrophage activity. Pinello KC, et al. Life Sci. 2006 (suma)

180. Antimicrobial activity of essential oils and carvacrol, and synergy of carvacrol and erythromycin, against clinical erythromycin-resistant Group A streptococci. Magi G, et al. Front Microbiol. 2015

181. Melaleuca alternifolia (Tea Tree) oil: a review of antimicrobial and other medicinal properties. Carson CF, et al. Clinical Microbiology Reviews 19(1) 50-6. 2015

182. Nicotine and health. Drug and therapeutics Bulletin. BMJ 2014

183. Betaine (N,N,N,-trimethylglycine) averts photo chemically-induced thrombosis in pial microvessels

in vivo and platelet aggregation in vitro. Nemmar A, et al. Exp Biol Med (Maywood). 2015

184. Curcumin enhanced cholesterol efflux by upregulating ABCA 1 expression through AMPK-SIRT 1=LXR alpha signaling in THP-1 macrophage-derived foam cells. Lin XL, et al. DNA Cell Biol. 2015 (a) Synthesis, characterization and anticancer activity of pluronic F-68 curcumin conjugate micelles. Cai Y, et al. Drug Deliv. 2015 (b)

   The beneficial role of curcumin on inflammation, diabetes and neurodegenerative disease: a recent update. Ghosh S, et al. Food Chem Toxicol. 2015 (c)

185. Comparative pharmacokinetics of rhein in normal and loperamide-induced constipated rays and microarray analysis of drug-metabolizing genes. Hou ML, et al. J Ethnopharmacol. 2014

186. Coriolus versicolor. American Cancer Society. Nov. 2008 (a)
   Efficacy of adjuvant immunochemotherapy with polysaccharide=k for patients with curative resections of gastric cancer. Oba K, et al. Cancer Immunol. 2007 (b) (turkey tail)

187. In vivo evaluation and safety profile evaluation of Arctostaphylos uva-ursi extract in rabbits. Saeed F, et al. Pak J Pharm Sci. 2014

188. Hyperactivity, concentration difficulties and impulsiveness improve during seven weeks' treatment with Valerian root and lemon balm extracts in primary school children. Gromball J, et al. Phytomedicine 2014

189. Vanillin protects human keratinocyte stem cells against ultraviolet B irradiation. Lee J, et al. Food Chem Toxicol. 204

190. Scientific evaluation of medicinal plant used for treatment of abnormal uterine bleeding by Avicenna. Mobli M, et al. Arch Gynecol Obstet. 2015 (vermicelle)

191. Novel neuroprotective effects of the aqueous extracts from Verbena officinalis Linn. Lai SW, et al. Neuropharmacology. 2006

192. Codex Guidelines for vitamin and mineral food supplements. Codex Alimentarius Commission/ United Nations. 2007

193. Chaste tree (vitex agnus-castus)-pharmacology and clinical indications. Wutte W, et al. Exp Clin Endocrinol Diabetes. 2003

194. Dehydration and endurance performance in competitive athletes. Goulet ED, et al. Nutr Rev. 2012 (a) (water)
   Common diagnosis and outcomes in elderly patients who present to the emergency depart-

ment with non-specific complaints. Quinn K, et al. CJEM. 2015 (b)

195. The antioxidant properties of isothiocyanate: a review. De Figueiredo SM, et al. Recent Pat Endocr Metab Immune Drug Discov. 2013 (watercress)

196. Isolation and characterization of feruloylated arabinoxylan oligosaccharides from the perennial cereal grain intermediate wheatgrass (Thinopyrum intermedium). Schendal PR, et al. Carbohydr Res. 2015

197. Systematic review and meta-analysis of human studies to support a quantitative recommendation for whole grain intake in relation to Type 2 diabetes. Chanson-Polle A, et al. PLos One. 2015

198. Evaluating the evidence for over the counter alternatives for relief of hot flashes in menopausal women. Kelley KW, et al. J Am Pharm Assoc. 2010 (wild yam)

199. Efficacy and safety of white willow bark (*Salix alba*) extracts. Shara M, et al. Phytother Res. 2015

200. Are one or two dangerous? Methylsalicylate exposure in toddlers. Davis JE, et al. J Emer Med. 2007. (wintergreen)

201. Hemorrhoids and varicose veins: a review of treatment options. Mackay D. Altern Med Rev. 2001 (witch hazel)

202. *Achillea millifolium* revisited: recent findings confirm traditional use. Benedek B, et al. Wien Med Wochenschr. 2007

203. A simple electrochemical method for the rapid estimation of antioxidant potentials of some selected medicinal plants. Amidi S, et al. Iran J Pharm Res. 2012 (yellow dock)

204. Maté: a risk factor for oral and oropharyngeal cancer. Goldenberg D, et al. Oral Oncol. 2002 (a) The positive effects of yerba mate (*Ilex paraguarensis*) in obesity. Gambero A, et al. Nutrients. 2015 (b)

    Antioxidant activity of polyphenols from green and toasted mate tea. Coentrão P de A, et al. Nat Prod Commun. 2011 (c) 206. Yohimbe: Medline Plus Supplements. NIH Nov. 2010

205. Zinc deficiency: has been known of for 40 years but ignored by global health organizations. Prasad A S, BMJ 2003

4

Specific Strategies for Disease Prevention

The following protocols contain disease prevention strategies. Some conventional treatments are mentioned where appropriate support for prevention is needed. Some alternative treatment strategies have been omitted as they are more effective for crisis management. The outline below highlights examples of some of the most common ailments encountered in modern industrialized communities. Identify and examine the one or ones that are of most concern or of particular susceptibility.

Infection

Prevention is achieved mainly by avoidance of situations in which infection is likely, such as exposure to bacterial, viral, fungal, parasitic vectors, and avoiding fatigue and stressors that reduce the immune system function.

1.   Keep hands clean/ personal hygiene (teeth x2/d; body bath).

2.   Keep surfaces clean (disinfectant, antiseptic).

3. Cover mouth and nose when sneezing or coughing/ avoid others who do not.

4. Avoid close contact with sick people.

5. Get immunizations: depending on exposure and age susceptibility: tetanus, chicken pox, measles, meningitis, shingles (>50), hepatitis, flu-influenza, pneumonia.

A healthy balanced diet that consists of good fats, low glycemic carbohydrates, mixed proteins, infection fighting fruit, vegetables, whole grains, lean meats, poultry, fish, beans, eggs, nuts, which are high in vitamins and minerals greatly boosts and maintains the immune system. Avoidance of saturated and trans fats and processed sugars (both *bacteria and cancer cells thrive on sugar*) is essential to good health.

With increasing age and indications of susceptibility to infections, one may consider taking one or two *immune system enhancers* three to five times a week.

Astragalus bark	Echinacea/goldenseal	Shiitake mushroom
Maitake mushroom	Agaricus blazei	Andrographis paniculata
Kelp	Cat's claw	Dandelion
Maca root	Moringa	Alfalfa

Common Plants and Fruit with Antibiotic Activity

Aloe vera	Barberry	Basil	Bergamot
Boldo	Comfrey	Calendula	Chamomile
Clove	Coconut oil	Cranberry	Echinacea
Garlic	Ginger	Goldenseal	Graviola
Guava	Hibiscus	Kalanchoe	Mace
Manuka honey	Marshmallow	Nutmeg	Olive leaf
Onion	Oregon grape root	Papaya	Thyme

Inflammation

Inflammation, such as that found in osteoarthritis, tendonitis, bursitis, gout, and many allergies is condition in which one or more body parts become hot, red, swollen, and painful due to injury, infection, or generalized immune system dysfunction. It often manifests with high blood levels of C-reactive protein, sedimentation rate, homocysteine levels, and IL-6, which are all toxic to the body. Some 80 percent of disease conditions involve inflammation either as cause or as effect. Affected persons have difficulty carrying on the activities of daily living (ADL) such as walking, eating, elimination, and sleeping. Frequently it is associated with obesity, poor diet, bad habits, and toxin exposure accumulation over a long period of time, and may be accompanied by hypertension, diabetes, heart disease, cancer, neurodegenerative disease, and/or arthritis. Including foods in the diet that reduce inflammation and avoiding foods that cause inflammation will greatly contribute to good health.

Anti-Inflammation Diet for All Inflammatory and Autoimmune Conditions

Omega 3 fish oils (wild salmon, tuna, sardines)	Iron (chickpeas, pinto beans, spinach)
Flaxseed oil, canola oil (cooking)	Extra virgin olive oil
Plant-based protein (beans, legumes, soy)	Ginger and turmeric daily
Antioxidants (fruit, berries, walnuts, seeds)	Green tea and Garlic
Vegetables (broccoli, collards, kale)	Vegetables (broccoli, collards, kale)
Fiber (whole wheat, cracked grains)	Vitamin B12 (corn, peanuts, wild rice, pasta)

Arthritis

(Osteoarthritis, tendonitis, bursitis, rheumatoid arthritis)

Osteoarthritis is inflammation of the joints, characterized by stiffness, decreased mobility, severe pain, and associated with trauma. It is chronic, progressive, and debilitating. Conventional treatment targeting the acute symptoms of pain and immobility lasts for short periods, requiring repetitive dosing, accompanied by serious side effects. A healthy functional well-regulated immune system will greatly reduce the risk of developing osteoarthritis at any age.

Preventive treatment goes after the biochemical causes. The goal is to avoid those things that lead to an excessive immune reaction or those things that lead to an excess suppression of the immune reaction and take in things that reduce or block the inflammatory process. A diet rich in anti-inflammation, anti-arthritis foods consists of cold water fish (omega-3 fatty acids and oils), avocado, and extra virgin olive oil as a main fat sources. Substitute animal-based proteins with plant-based proteins like soy, beans, quinoa, wild rice, hummus, and peanut butter. Reduce milk products and use yogurt for calcium instead. Increase the intake of organic fruit and vegetables for the antioxidant effect, and eat more fiber, garlic, walnuts and flaxseed for additional omega 3 supplementation. Drink one-half your body weight in ounces of pure water daily.

Avoid all trans and saturated fats (margarine, vegetable shortening, partially hydrogenated, and deep fried foods), cooking oil that "smokes," fast foods, animal fats (red meat, poultry skin, egg yolks, whole milk dairy products), white sugar, excess alcohol, refined carbohydrates (sodas and high sugar pastries), white flour, and all tobacco products.

Supplementation: With early symptoms, you may take glucosamine/chondroitin, 1,500 mg a day, and/or SAMe, which help to build cartilage. A multivitamin with MSM, vitamin D, K, and selenium would also be effective. The two natural anti-inflammation products that are most effective are turmeric and ginger on a daily basis, in soups, stews, teas, powder, or capsules. Recommended botanicals for reducing inflammation are cats claw 250 to 1,000mg/d; Boswellia, 400 to 1,200mg/d; devil's claw, 600 to 1,200mg/d; and guggul 500 to 1,000mg daily. Bromelain is an enzyme in fresh pineapples that will reduce internal inflammation. Capsaicin in cayenne pepper when applied topically will decrease nerve pain. A poultice of lobelia, mullein, slippery elm, and cayenne can be applied for relief of swollen joints. The high levels of flavonoids in cherries offer some relief for joint pain. Plants like starchy roots, leafy greens, soy and foods from animal bones, skin, and connective tissue (soups and stews), are rich in hyaluronic acid and have been shown to prevent and even reverse the effects of osteoarthritis.

Full range of motion (ROM) exercises should be done regularly with stretching and yoga poses for flexibility. Inactivity will guarantee progression to immobility. Walk thirty minutes a day, three to five times a week. Aerobics for cardiovascular health, biking, running, and swimming should maintain ROM and not increase pain. Regular physical activity stimulates the immune system and reduces stress hormone levels. Apply heat before and cool after exercising.

Traditional Chinese medicine offers acupuncture that is especially effective for neck and low back pain. A homeopathic arthritic gel and arthritic formula and rubefacients with salicylates for the joints are available. Magnetic therapy may benefit the hip and knees.

Rheumatoid arthritis is associated with autoimmune factors often related to social, emotional, and sleep-deprivation issues. Aside from the psychological approaches, the prevention and treatment regimen for both conditions is the same: increase anti-inflammation measures and avoid pro-inflammation causes.

Gout is the severe inflammation mainly of the first metatarsal joint of the foot (big toe) that results from excessively high levels of uric acid in the blood. Due to overproduction, abnormal processing, or under-elimination of uric acid by the kidneys, it is usually accompanied by excessive intake of purine-rich foods like red meat and heavy sauces. It is manifested by severe pain, restricted ambulation, and may lead to joint destruction and deterioration of other organs. It has also been found in the joints of the fingers and other toes.

Conventional treatment is with allopurinol and colchicine for the uric acid and NSAIDS, corticosteroids, ACTH, probenecid, and sulfinpyrazone for the inflammatory pain, plus serious side effects.

Prevention and treatment is first through *avoidance* of purine-rich meats (lamb, beef, game, venison), increased water intake to dilute and neutralize the acids, reduction in alcohol intake, especially of spirits and high tannin wines, and weight reduction. Drink apple cider vinegar , one teaspoon in a cup of water, three times a day to cut the uric acid; eat pectin (apples, cherries, blackberry juice) and take turmeric and ginger, one teaspoon each in cooked food or teas, daily. Cayenne ointment and tincture of lobelia with apple cider vinegar may be applied to the affected joint to relieve the pain. Detoxification two to three times a week may be done with skullcap, valerian, and yarrow tea or with the more common apple cider vinegar, lemon, and olive oil combination of one tablespoon each three times a day.

Allergy is the "rage" of the disease menu for the twenty-first century. Mild to severe "reactions" of the immune system to external or internal substances, like food, pollutants, medications, and toxins, occur when the body is exposed to an allergen that it deems foreign and a threat. Controversy exists as to the causes, but the increase in C-section births in which the immune system does not get the chance to experience the natural birth event, the increase in exposure to toxic influences, and the obsession with cleanliness in the early years, all contribute to underdeveloped and errantly directed immunity. Conventional treatments address acute attacks with epinephrine, antihistamines, and steroids; and chronicity with elimination and low protein diets, extensive allergy testing and avoidance. Heavy attention is given to gluten and milk as the awful culprits that must be avoided by all means possible.

Prevention and treatment is directed to building and improving the function of the immune system without the suppression that leaves the individual totally dependent on medications…until they outgrow it or it goes away. Basic immune/allergy reconstruction consists of increase in antioxidant-rich fruit and vegetables (berries and cherries have flavonoids that regulate the immune response); omega-3 fish oils (wild-caught salmon), and fresh-ground flaxseed on cereal or wild rice two to three times a week. Increase water intake to keep passages moist and flush out the system. Daily vitamin C, bee pollen, and quercetin-rich foods are good immune system regulators. For acute attacks or bites, noni leaf, calendula, or tea tree oil applications act as cortisone or Benadryl. Fried-dried stinging nettle and butterbur are both as good as antihistamines, yet without the drowsiness.

For chronic recurrences and reconstruction of immunity, acupuncture decreases stress response, homeopathy with arnica, and A*llium cepa* (garlic) are especially effective in young children and hypnosis in adults. All are evidence-based and scientifically proven to be safe and effective.

Botanicals for allergies include fenugreek, devil's claw, Echinacea (best for acute attacks), the Chinese Fo-ti, hydrangea, kudzu vine, *Picrorhiza kurroa* (asthma) and yerba santa.

Autoimmune Diseases

Lupus erythematosus is a collection of diseases in which a hyperactive immune system attacks normal body tissues, namely kidneys, joints, skin, blood cells, heart, and lungs, severely impairing function. Conventional treatment is with immunosuppressive drugs like hydrochloroquine, corticosteroids, and the new synthetic belimubab. The side effects are considerable. *Avoidance* of foods high in saturated and polyunsaturated fats, like sunflower and corn oil, red meat, sodas, all processed like white sugar, rice, bread, and canned foods. Alfalfa sprouts are particularly dangerous as they contain L-canavanine, which stimulates the immune system to trigger inflammation. It should be noted that some autoimmune diseases like amyotropic lateral sclerosis (ALS) have been associated with exposure to external toxins like formaldehyde inhalation.

Prevention should proceed by using a diet rich in omega-3 fatty acids like alpha linolenic acid (ALA), lignans (canola oil, dark leafy greens), flaxseed oil (EPA), fresh fruit and vegetables, like vitamin C rich broccoli, kale, and cabbage, plus kiwi and citrus for strong antioxidant DNA cell repair, as well as vitamin E rich egg yolks, milk, nuts, whole grains for nerve and endothelium cell repair. The natural anti-inflammation supplements, turmeric, and ginger, should be taken daily. Exercise in the form of aerobics, swimming, walking, should be done regularly, to stimulate the effects of endorphins and other endogenous healing hormones.

Multiple sclerosis is a progressive central nervous system autoimmune disease where the inflammatory cells attack the myelin sheath of the neurons resulting in disruption of nerve signals and destruction of the brain, optic nerve, and spinal cord. The cause is multifactorial in that both genetic and environmental (virus?) triggers may be involved. Women between the ages of twenty to forty are more likely to contract MS than are men. Avoidance of toxins is very important, such as cooking in aluminum foil, canned and processed foods, and eating non-organic foods grown with pesticides and fertilizers. Conventional treatment is with potent corticosteroids to achieve intense immunosuppression to delay progression and reduce flare-ups, but this will also leave the patient without viable immunity and highly susceptible to superinfections.

Prevention involves a change from a diet of bad food to good food. Reduce protein intake to 10 percent (use plant-based proteins), eliminate milk (get calcium from vegetables and yogurt), use extra virgin olive oil as the main fat, and increase omega-3 intake, like salmon, sardines, tuna, fish oils, walnuts, flaxseed and soy foods, five grams daily. This should give added antioxidant DNA repair and healing and prevention of nerve cell breakdown. Supplement with ginger and turmeric daily for inflammation control and CoQ10 30mg two to three times a week for cell regulation. Consider bee pollen, which is rich in vitamins, proteins, carbohydrates, minerals, and enzymes to boost the immune system and build resistance. Lecithin helps to repair myelin sheath damage. Exercise with light aerobics and yoga, four to five times a week to keep the circulation healthy. Seek positive stress control through mind-body, homeopathy, magnetic therapy, meditation, and craniosacral techniques.

Other autoimmune diseases include dermatomyositis, glomerulonephritis, myasthenia, gravis, pemphigoid, Sjogren's syndrome, vitiligo, Wegener's granulomatosis, scleroderma, psoriasis, polymyositis, some uveitis, and some thyroiditis...which may respond to prevention measures as well.

A healthy immune system has regulatory T cells, killer T cells, with a complement system of defensins and phagocytes with immunological memory that react to stressors by destroying the invaders, neutralizing harmful reactive oxygen species and free radicals, clean up, and maintain good "health." Quality sleep and relaxation, regular exercise, a healthy balanced diet, and effective stress reduction are basic requirements.

Specific Immune System Enhancers for Cancer Prevention

Astragalus root	Echinacea	Maitake mushroom
Shiitake mushroom	Goldenseal	Turkey tail
Kelp	Hydrangea	Cat's claw
Dandelion root	Maca root	Alfalfa
Agaricus blazei	Andrographicus paniculata	Vitamin C

Cancer Prevention

A diagnosis of cancer is one of the most feared events in human existence. Definitive detection can be made when there are a billion cancer cells or more in a given tissue. If there are only a few million or less, the cancer may be undetectable by standard tests but is still present. One in three diagnosed cases will progress. Early diagnosis and treatment as a viable strategy is well known. Treatment with surgery, radiation, and chemotherapy, though often successful, can be accompanied with serious side effects. *Cancer prevention to keep the cell numbers well below detection is a more effective defense.*

Causes: Every person has cancer cells. All cancers are multifactorial and result from a combination of heredity, environmental factors, and bad luck. Prevention can be instituted by eliminating the trigger mechanisms like environmental factors and lifestyle changes that are linked with the mutations that drive the cell divisions. A poor lifestyle and faulty genetics increases cancer risk while a healthy lifestyle and normal genetics results in well-being. So why does Mr. A who has never smoked, get lung cancer, and Mr. B, who smoked three packs a day since he was twenty, does not. The answer lies in the presence of intrinsic biochemical and bio-physiological systems that play a role in determining, which signaling mechanisms to and from cells will be turned on and off. Their status is determined by a combination of genetic and environmental factors. The status of the immune system is a very strong determinant of when, where, and how factors of expression, proliferation, and destruction are manifested. A functional immune system keeps cancer cells in check. When *the immune system* weakens in the presence of active risk factors, affected cells fail to die on schedule, continue to proliferate into "tumors," which use up all the nutrients leaving normal cells to die prematurely and organs to fail. The main causes of impaired immunity besides genetic predisposition are nutritional and hormonal deficiencies, poor lifestyle choices involving obesity and inflammation, environmental toxins, some medical treatments including chemotherapy, radiation, and some prescription drugs. The *stress* created by the knowledge of the ordeal, low survival statistics, side effects of conventional treatments and prospects of financial obligations and potential ruin, can seriously affect the outcome. The release of excess stress hormones can only be detrimental to the containment of cancer cells. Cancer is a disease of the body, mind, and spirit. Using positivity to dispense with anger, melancholy, revenge, and depression will always help.

The following is a brief list of some common carcinogens the exposure to which greatly increases the risk of cancer.

Environmental Carcinogens

Endocrine disrupting chemicals	Pesticides (DDT, DEET, Atrazine)	Glyphosates (weed-killer)
Fertilizers (nitrates)	Phthalates (plastic containers)	Bisphenol A (BPA) can linings

Polyvinyl chloride (PVC) piping	Styrene (food packaging)	GMO's (genetic modification)
Processed meat (sodium nitrite)	Perfluroctanic acid mw popcorn	Zeranol (hormone to cattle)
Bovine growth hormone	4-methyl imidazole (soda coloring)	heavy metals (cadmium, nickel, cyanide, arsenic)
Cleaning supplies (dioxin)	Lindane (y-BHC)	benzene hexachloride (a-BHC)
Cigarette smoke (hydrocarbons)	asbestos	formaldehyde

Chemotherapy as a treatment for cancer poisons all cells immediately and causes mutations in cancer cells, some good, others bad, in the long term. Extensive surgery can spread cancer cells to other sites (metastasis). Radiation burns, creates scars, damages healthy cells, and harms the immune system. The treatments may leave the body open to fatal super infections. Some approved prescription medications, associated with cancer in rodents, are still under investigation for their link to cancer in humans.

Natural remedies for nausea induced by chemotherapy:

Ginger tea,raw,lozenges	Cannabis sativa (THC)	Fennel tea	Kudzu/ arrowroot tea
Licorice (DGL)	Multivitamin (Propax)	relaxation techniques	exercise

Natural remedies for burns and pain induced by radiation:

Granoderma	Spirulina	Aloe vera gel (apply)	Caraway seed tea

After chemotherapy and/or radiation:

Green tea	Vitamin C	Antioxidant foods
High protein foods	Alpha lipoic acid	Coconut water

Cancer-Associated Prescription Medications

Hormone replacement Therapy (estrogens)	Omeprazole (Prilosec for heartburn)	Spironolactone (for high blood pressure)	Elidel and Protopic (for eczema)
Humira, Cimzia, Enbrel, Remicade injections for rheumatoid arthritis	statins and fibrates for cholesterol control	Simvastatin and ezetimibe for cholesterol control	Diabetic drugs with pioglitazone and/or glimepiride

Cancer-Causing Foods

Red meat (well-done/charred)	Sugar (white and brown)	Diet aspartame, MSG, saccharin
Acidic foods	White flour (processed)	Treated fruit (trucked for miles)

Farmed fish (grain-fed, Vit D)	Hydrogenated oils, transfats	Alcohol (DNA damage)
Baked goods (acrylamides)	Sodas, soft drinks (coloring)	Smoked/salted heterocyclic amines)

Cancer cells thrive in an acid medium full of sugar. Avoid overcooked foods with nitrites, nitrates, sulfates, chlorides, bromates, that are products of chemical breakdowns, as well as high-glycemic sugars, like glucose, aldose, sucrose, and synthetic high fructose corn syrup.

Prevention: A healthy functional immune system is essential to preventing and fighting off cancer cells. Fifty percent (50%) of cancers are preventable by making the right lifestyle choices. In addition to avoidance of cancer-causing products, some foods, and plants contain chemicals that can prevent cancer cells from becoming dominant and destroy them in the early stages. These "good" chemicals that contribute to the balance of hormones and vitamins in the immune system are found in whole foods in higher and more natural concentrations than in supplements. Large amounts of either would have to be taken in order for the evidence-based effect to occur. However, a diet high in fiber, low in fat, and laden with cancer preventing foods plus a strict avoidance of cancer causing environmental toxins, will reduce the risk and susceptibility of contracting cancer.

Cancer Preventing Foods and Botanicals

Broccoli, cabbage, cauliflower	Leafy greens (spinach, kale)	Green tea (catechins)
Mushrooms (shiitake)	Chamomile (apigenin)	Brazil nuts (selenium)
Artichokes (salvestrol)	Tomatoes (lycopene)	Grapes/ red wine (resveratrol)
Legumes (beans, peas)	Berries (anthrocyanosides)	Flaxseed (antioxidants)
Garlic, onions, chives, leeks	Olive oil (oleuropein)	Fruit (polyphenols)
Tangerine (Vit C, nobilitin)	Potatoes (chlorogenic acid)	Cereals, whole grains (fiber)
Soy (isoflavones)	Vitamin D and E	seaweed (kelp, dulse)
Almonds	Apples/ apple cider vinegar	Burdock root
Carrots (carotenoids)	Celery	Horseradish
Lentils	Millet	Sesame oil
Orange peels	Parsley	Radishes
Rhubarb	Stinging nettle	Watercress
Anamú	Basil	Ginger
Lemongrass	Goatweed	Cayenne pepper
Rosemary	Moringa	Turmeric

Keep your weight down to normal or at least less than BMI 25 (body mass index). Obesity is strongly linked to inflammation which is associated with cancer cell growth.

Include a high percentage of vegetables in the diet (80 percent); add nuts, seeds, whole grains, fruit, cooked fish, skinless poultry, and lots of legumes, especially as you age. Five servings of fruit and vegetables a day reduces cancer risk by 35 to 50 percent through their strong antioxidant activity.

Get plenty of sleep to maintain circadian rhythm and regular DNA repair.

Avoid stress in the form of anger, bitterness, grudges, as this will seriously affect levels of serotonin, GABA, 5-Tryptophan and glutamic acid necessary for regular brain function.

Physical activity on a regular basis is needed to ensure adequate oxygenation of cells and tissues. Exercise is positively associated with reduced risk of breast, colon, and endometrial cancers. Possible pathways involve insulin resistance, growth factors, release of steroid hormones, and better immune function. Physical activity is linked to increased cancer survival.

Drink more water. Cancer cells thrive at high levels of retained carbon dioxide (CO_2). Drink alkaline purified water to deprive cancer cells of growth promoting acid. *Avoid* distilled water or carbonated sodas.

Starve cancer cells by cutting off their energy source. Refined sugar and sugar substitutes like aspartame, table salt with color additives, whole milk producing mucus in the GI tract, red meat, high caffeine, distilled water, and all

junk food, create high acidity on which cancer cells thrive
must be *avoided*. It is safer to use honey, stevia, agave, or
molasses; sea salt or Braggs amino salt; unsweetened soy
milk; alkaline fish and chicken; and green tea.

Do not put plastic water bottles in the freezer as they may
release dioxin upon melting. No plastic in the microwave.
Use wax paper to cover approved plates and containers.

Phytochemicals that block DNA oxidative damage and delay cancer onset:

Indole-3-carbinol	Epigallocatechins	Curcumin	Isoflavones
Folic acid	Allicin/ allyl sulfides	Carotenoids	Flavonoids
Chlorophyll	Isothiocyanates	Polyphenols	Protease inhibitors
Organosulfides	Inositol phosphates	Terpenes	Quercetin
Acids (ellagic, caffeic...)	Benzaldehyde	Coumarins	Dithiolthiones
Germanium	Genistein	Glutathione	Glycosides
Lecithin	Lignans	Phytosterols	Saponins
Sulforaphane	Tannins	Quinones	Limonene

These phytochemicals found in fruit, herbs, vegetables,
and spices, help to prevent, neutralize, and destroy cancer
cells by inhibition of the proteins required for their growth
and reproduction, direct killing by DNA inhibition
(cytotoxic), indirectly by antioxidant scavenging of free
radical to prevent DNA damage and stimulate repair
in healthy cells and by destruction or blockage of their

enzymes needed for function. Though the amounts required for a measureable effect are large, loading up with four to five servings a day is a particularly good idea.

If and when prevention is sought or cancer is suspected, the following supplements are recommended...the first six groups, daily, the last six, two to three times a week.

Must-Take for Cancer Prevention and Treatment

Green tea	Turmeric and Ginger	Green leafy vegetables
Omega 3 (flaxseed, fish oils)	Garlic and Onions	Astragalus root
Coenzyme Q 10 90-120 mg	Graviola (soursop)	Moringa oleifera
Melatonin 3 mg	Milk thistle/ dandelion 200mg	Figs and apricots

Exercise: Cancer cells love a carbon dioxide environment. Get rid of carbon dioxide and oxygenize your body with regular physical activity, deep breathing techniques, and in some cases, ozone therapy. Regular physical activity has a positive association with lowered risk of cancer.

Specific Prevention

Cancer of the Blood

Leukemia is a group of cancers in which the white blood cells increase in number, size, and configuration. The exact cause is largely unknown, but points to errors in control of normal cell division and breakdown in the immune system function. Risk factors include exposure to chemicals like benzene, ionizing radiation, chemotherapy, viruses, which may lead to genetic mutations and impaired immunity. It may be ironic as the conventional treatment is with chemotherapy and radiation.

Prevention aims at promoting healthy blood components, especially B cells to produce antibodies against infections and T cells to kill invasive foreign bodies directly, with vitamin B6 and B12, which help to lower the levels of homocysteine (toxin), chlorophyll, folates, and iron (in beets, lentils, kidney beans, prunes, green vegetables) to increase red blood cells. The phytochemicals in garlic (*allicin*), olive leaf extract, milk thistle, and licorice root all reduce the rate of cancer cell replication, while green tea, turmeric, and *Hedyotis diffusa* all promote apoptosis (*programmed cell death*). Aloe vera purifies the blood, and panax ginseng both prevents and destroys leukemia cells. Despite being natural cancer cell killers, such large amounts of these products are required for a desired effect that the blood thinning side effects should be taken into account. Evidence exists that tangerines, with tangiritin and noilitin, can inhibit the formation of leukemia cells.

Hodgkin's lymphoma starts in the lymph nodes in the neck, underarm, and chest, spreads node to node then later to the blood stream. Accounting for some 95 percent of cases, cancer lymph cells are larger than normal lymphocytes, and all are malignant. Non-Hodgkin's lymphoma also starts in the lymph nodes then spreads to the spleen and bone marrow.

Multiple myeloma is cancer of the plasma cells of the blood, in which the proteins break down due to poor diet, excessive alcohol intake, overload of cigarette toxins, particularly cadmium and nickel, exposure to air and water pollutants, molds (mycotoxins), new plastics, chemical air fresheners, harsh cleaning agents, and inadequate sleep, all contributing to a dysfunctional immune system. *Avoid* cooked food and frozen drinks from BPA plastic containers. Do not cook food at high temperatures (fried) to reduce exposure to carcinogenic acrylamides. Conventional treatment is mainly with chemotherapy (thalidomide, bisphosphonates) to kill fast-growing cells, massive doses of corticosteroids to suppress immunity, radiation, and stem cell transplantation, none of which have very good results.

Prevention strategies for all blood and lymphatics consist of primary avoidance of toxins and maintaining a healthy immune system. Regular detoxifications with lemon juice, apple cider vinegar, and olive oil mixture, one teaspoon daily for three days a week; a balanced diet of whole foods with full complement of vitamins and minerals to build up red and white blood cells and platelets; plenty of clean drinking water; monthly blood purification with burdock, goldenseal, dandelion, or sarsaparilla; and one or two immune system enhancers like astragalus root, maitake medicinal mushrooms, hydrangea, kelp, or maca root are recommended.

Cancer of the Central Nervous System

Brain cancer is mainly related to genetic factors in children (Turcot syndrome with abnormal cells and polyps and neurofibromatosis with nodular fibrous growths on the skin and in the brain), radiation to the head, age (more common in the over sixty-five age group), HIV infection, cigarette smoking, and environmental toxins (chemicals associated with oil refineries, embalming chemicals, and rubber processing).

Prevention can be pursued through a ketogenic diet of high fat, high protein, and extremely low carbohydrates in which the body then produces ketones instead of glucose. The brain can get energy from ketones, but cancer cells only use glucose. Other cancer prevention foods include garlic, broccoli, berries, tomatoes, green tea, whole grains, turmeric, dark, leafy, green vegetables, beans and grapes, all containing phytochemicals with potent antioxidant and cytotoxic activity.

Cancer of the Skin

Basal cell carcinoma, squamous cell carcinoma, and malignant melanoma are three of the most common skin cancers all associated with excessive exposure and damage to the DNA of skin cells leading to abnormal growth by ultraviolet radiation (UVA long wavelength and UVB short wavelength) from the sun. Risk factors include individuals with fair skin, freckles, and red hair, with vitamin D and melanin deficiency. Older individuals with normally aged skin cells are also more susceptible. Though the pigment melanin is protective, anyone can get skin cancer given the length and time of exposure and functional condition of the immune system. In general, the less melanin results in the less protection and higher risk for skin cancer. More exposure at the equator or tropics on bright white sandy beaches at altitude with less cloud protection and in tanning booths, all types, with intermittent intense doses, also increases the risk. Those with exposure to heavy metal toxins like arsenic (*in well water and pesticides*), coal tar, paraffin, and certain oils, those with numerous or large moles, or with rough scaly skin plaques (*actinic keratosis*), and after radiation treatment are also at high risk. Smokers, those with human papilloma virus warts, HIV infection, under treatment with large doses of corticosteroids and subsequent weakened immune system are more susceptible to skin cancer.

Prevention consists mainly of avoidance. Stay away from exposure to intense radiation from 10:00 AM to 2:00 PM when the sun is at its highest. Avoid tanning beds, especially if carrying any of the above risk factors. Sunscreen of no less than SPF (sun protection factor) 15 in temperate zones and SPF 30 in tropical zones are recommended for the average fair-skinned individual. If the skin normally "reddens" in twenty minutes, then SPF will take five hours to redden and SPF 30 may take eight to ten hours. However, the higher numbers are only slightly more protective. The best sunscreen is a broad spectrum combination of organic to absorb and inorganic to reflect and scatter UV radiation, with coconut oil and/or aloe vera to counteract the drying effects of the sun on the skin. Clothing consisting of long pants, shirt sleeves, and a hat with a wide brim will also offer protection.

Cancer of the Lung

Lung cancer is the leading cause of death by cancer in both men and women in the USA. The main causes are due to the inhalation of irritants and carcinogens leading to uncontrolled growth of abnormal cells that line the air passages, which divide rapidly to form fast-growing tumors with a high frequency of metastasis. Cigarette smoke contains over seventy toxic chemicals such as nicotine, tars like polycyclic aromatic hydrocarbons, and nitrosamine-butanone, and heavy metals like arsenic, cadmium, and nickel, cause mutations in oncogenes and tumor suppressor genes that allows for oxidative stress damage and subsequent cancer cell formation. Cigar and pipe smoking cause more cancer than not smoking. Younger onset age of cigarette smoking is at higher risk due to the time available for cumulative effects. Second-hand smoke or environmental tobacco smoke is exhaled smoke that is then secondarily inhaled by another person, is a serious health hazard and auxiliary cause of death. Individuals with a weakened immune system such as HIV, AIDS, or on immunosuppressant drugs, autoimmune disease like rheumatoid arthritis, a family history of susceptibility, women with the estrogen receptor breast cancer gene (BRCA 1 and 2), smokers taking vitamin A (beta-carotene), exposure to radon gas, asbestos, silica, and diesel exhaust are at higher risk.

Prevention is primarily through avoidance of exposure to known carcinogens. Stop smoking. A diet high in fresh fruit and vegetables with strong antioxidant activity of removal of harmful reactive oxygen species and free radicals, such as vitamins A, C, and E, plus flavonoids is recommended. Large amounts of aspirin, which reduce inflammation, have an indirect effect, but the side effects neutralize the benefits.

Women's Cancer

Breast cancer is the leading cause of cancer death in women in the USA. The risk factors include over age fifty, positive family history, presence of the genes BRCA 1 and 2, increased estrogen after menopause (like HRT and E2P4 therapy), post-menopausal obesity, sedentary lifestyle, and exposure to environmental carcinogens (cigarette smoking and endocrine disruptor chemicals). There are 216 chemicals that induce cancer in animals. Those associated with human breast cancer are industrial solvents, pesticides like atrazine and phthalates, various dyes, gasoline and diesel exhausts, certain cosmetic ingredients, chlorinated drinking water, acrylamide in French fries, and 1, 4-dioxane in shampoos. Though all women may be exposed to various degrees, some will be more susceptible depending on status of the immune system and levels of antioxidants and their ability to repair damaged DNA.

Prevention should begin with the awareness that the presence of genetic markers, high levels of estrogen particularly after menopause and exposure to high levels of carcinogens will increase the risk. Clean the home and remove as many toxins as possible. Reduce *exposure* to xenoestrogens like those found in pesticides, industrial pollutants, hormone residues in meat, poultry and dairy products, and radiation (frequent chest X-rays, mammograms). Note close relatives with breast cancer and consider genetic testing, counseling, and discussion of personal drug therapy or surgery.

Eat foods to counter the effects of estrogen: soy products, olive oil, canola (monounsaturated fats), cruciferous vegetables (broccoli, cabbage, cauliflower, kale, radishes, watercress, bok choy) hormone-free, organic meats, dairy, and poultry. Take in fruits and vegetables (antioxidants) on a daily basis that are known to reduce the incidence of premenopausal breast CA, green tea instead of coffee, omega-3, and extra virgin olive oil. Replace estrogens with natural phytoestrogens, like soy and tofu, which are rich in isoflavones and inositol phosphates. Get folates from dark leafy greens like spinach, kale, red cabbage, romaine lettuce, and lean red meat, which have carotenoids and are also cytotoxic.

(See appendix for a more complete list of anticancer foods.)

Consider taking a multivitamin with vitamin D (at least 1000IU /day), plus daily sunshine if possible. Supplements with seaweed (kelp) are cytotoxic to cancer cells. Shiitake mushrooms with conjugated linoleic acid will inhibit the enzyme aromatase which makes estrogen, plus it stimulates the immune system. Calcium D-Glucarate prevents estrogenic cancers by detoxifying carcinogens and has been shown to reduce breast cancer in rats. The antioxidant, co-enzyme Q10, assists in the production of energy (ATPs) in the inner membrane of the mitochondria effects on immune system and protects normal tissues from free radical damage caused by conventional cancer treatment. Melatonin, the pineal hormone associated with diurnal rhythm regulation, has strong anti-estrogenic effects and is also protective against uterine cancer.

Exercising on a regular basis for a minimum of thirty minutes a day is protective of cancer, builds immune system, releases beneficial endorphin hormones, and regulates the stress hormone, cortisol. Manage the weight. Post-menopausal women who gained eleven to eighteen pounds had a higher risk than those who gained only four pounds.

Excess weight is directly associated with inflammation, which plays an integral part in the onset and progression of cancer.

Over the age of forty, early detection through self-examinations as well as an *annual* breast exam and/or scheduled mammograms is recommended.

The mind-body approach to preventive medicine is directed mainly to the reduction of stress. Yoga, hypnosis, biofeedback, meditation, guided imagery, music therapy, and breathing exercises, will reduce stress, provide comfort and improve the immune system function by increasing good natural killer cells and the number of peripheral blood lymphocytes needed to prevent and combat infection and inflammation.

Ovarian cancer can occur in any of three layers: the outer epithelial (most common), middle stromal, hormone-producing layer, and the inner germ cell, egg-producing layer. The highest risk is in the fifty- to sixty-year-old age group. The genetic risk is similar to that of breast cancer with the BRCA 1 and 2 gene markers, and associated HRT (estrogen hormone replacement therapy), long term, and in large doses. Those who experience the onset of menstruation before age twelve, menopause after age fiifty-two, never pregnant, smokers, using IUD, and a history of polycystic ovary syndrome, are also at greater risk. A high intake of processed meat, fried foods (acrylamides), and milk protein (more than three glasses a day), which increases levels of insulin-like growth factor, may fuel cancer cells and increase the risk.

Prevention through the use of birth control pills for five or more years has been shown. One should be aware of other side effects, like an increase in the risk of breast cancer. If a positive family history is present, then genetic counselling with possible tubal ligation and/or hysterectomy surgeries may be indicated. A natural diet rich in cruciferous vegetables like cauliflower and broccoli, have been linked to a definite reduction in colon, breast, ovarian, bladder, and prostate cancers. Cucumbers contain lignans, which have direct cytotoxic activity against ovarian, breast, uterine, and prostate cancers. Cold water fish with omega 3 fatty acids reduced risk of ovarian cancer by 25 percent. Micronutrients from plant based foods like ginger, ginkgo biloba, green tea (*Chinese women drinking oolong, green, and black tea were 70 percent less likely to develop ovarian cancer*), and flaxseed are rich in antioxidants and contribute to preventing cancer cells from forming. These must be taken in large amounts of up to eight to ten servings a day, for the maximum effect. Regular aspirin has been shown to reduce the risk through its reduction of inflammation, but not NSAIDS or acetaminophen.

Uterine cancer is associated with an imbalance in the ratio between estrogen and progesterone (high E and low P), which leads to a thickening of the lining of the uterus and a proliferation of cancer cells. Risk factors include increased age, taking estrogen therapy after menopause, radiation to treat another cancer, a high total number of menstrual cycles (starting before age twelve and ending after age fifty-two), obesity (*as fat tissue can change androgen hormones into estrogens thereby contributing to the imbalance*), a high-fat diet, polycystic ovarian disease, and diabetes.

Prevention may include taking melatonin (3 to 10 mg) a pineal hormone, diurnal rhythm regulator, and antioxidant that reduces estrogen production by blocking the enzyme, aromatase at the receptor site. Taking melatonin if on Tamoxifen for post-breast cancer is especially effective. Pregnancy in itself will protect against high estrogen levels as the progesterone in naturally increased. Use of an intrauterine device (IUD) and birth control pills will also reduce the risk.

Gastrointestinal Cancer

Stomach cancer is the second leading cause of cancer-related death in the world (after lung cancer). The risk factors include oxidative stress and DNA damage to the mucosal cells of the inner lining, by excess acids, Helicobacter pylori bacterial infection, bad eating habits leading to frequent indigestion, chronic inflammation, and absorption of the chemicals of processed food and smoking.

Prevention is by improvement of eating habits to include foods high in antioxidants that prevent and repair damaged lining cells. Foods high in carotenoids, *red, green, and yellow vegetables*, with lycopene and lutein, are especially adept at keeping the stomach lining functional and healthy. Kelp, probiotics, and legumes with protease inhibitors, aid digestion, and are cytotoxic to early tumor cells. Chamomile tea with apigenin is specific for inhibition of Helicobacter pylori bacteria and prevention of gastric cancers.

Colon cancer is associated with physical and emotional oxidative stress triggering genetic mutations in high energy cells of the mucosal lining. Chronic irritants from heavy fatty and processed meats like bacon, sausage, hot dogs, ham, cold cuts), carcinogens from smoking, environmental pollutants, depressed immunity from high alcohol intake, age and stress-related hormonal changes in post-menopausal women, excess body weight, inactivity, presence of polyps, and poor metabolism all contribute to the high risk of colon cancer.

Prevention: 33 percent of colon cancers can be avoided by adopting a high-fiber, low-fat diet, that includes beans, lentils, legumes, whole grains, fruit (*antioxidants and antiplatelet activity*), and vegetables up to five servings a day. Whole food and supplements with calcium and folic acid such as in fortified cereals, contribute protective micronutrients. Apricots, beets, blueberries, cherries, cabbage, cantaloupe, carrots, chili peppers with capsaicin, plums, figs, garlic, grapefruit, grapes, lemons, oranges, and olive oil are all protective and preventive. Herbs and spices with terpenes (isoprenoids) and selenium, like Brazil nuts, are directly cytotoxic to colon cancer cells.

Physical activity such as regular and routine walking of thirty minutes a day, five days a week, promotes bowel health, is healing and preventive. Aspirin in low doses appears to increase survival rates for colon, rectal, and esophageal cancers through its action of reducing inflammation in the bowels, reducing abnormal clotting, repairing damaged blood vessels, and enabling the immune system to recognize and disable abnormal circulating tumor cells. Be aware that high doses and prolonged use may damage the stomach lining.

Liver cancer cells grow into tumors from mutations due to mistakes for chemical detoxification processes. The most common risk factor (50 percent) is cirrhosis due to alcohol abuse. Other high risk is associated with chronic infection due to hepatitis B and C, fatty liver disease, obesity, diabetes, hereditary conditions like hemochromatosis and Wilson's disease, and exposure to aflatoxins, poisons produced by molds growing on poorly stored products like corn and peanuts.

Prevention is by maintaining a healthy liver through foods with protective properties, like artichokes, with salvestrol, cranberries, with ursolic acid, quercetin, and other compounds that inhibit the proliferation of hepatocellular carcinoma, and soy, with genistein that inhibits liver cancer cells through potent antioxidant activity.

Pancreatic cancer arises in two types of cells: one that produces hormones (endocrine) and the other that produces enzymes (exocrine). Risk factors include age over fifty-five, individuals with genetic mutations associated with BRCA 2 breast cancer gene, excessive alcohol intake and cigarette smoking with cumulative damage, chronic pancreatitis (inflammation) associated with H. pylori infection, obesity, diabetes, and cirrhosis.

Prevention is directed to reducing inflammation. The consumption of fresh fruit and vegetables, especially those with high vitamin C and carotenoid antioxidant content, is protective. Plant-based foods that inhibit COX 2 expression, like ginger, turmeric, cayenne pepper, licorice, kelp, flaxseed and goldenseal are protective.

Genitourinary System

Kidney and bladder cancers arise readily from chronic irritants that accumulate in the urine, damage the mucosal lining and promote the formation of cancer cells, which grow rapidly due to the favorable acidic, high-glycemic environment. Risk factors include over age forty, exposure to arsenic in drinking water, factory smelters, chemicals used in dyes, rubber, textiles, and paint products, radiation, parasitic infection with schistosomiasis, chronic cystitis, and some on diabetic medications with the chemicals, pioglitazone, and glimepiride like metformin and actos.

Prevention is through the promotion of DNA methylation with antioxidant flavonoids like cranberries, tomatoes, grapes, spinach, broccoli, and legumes, with 2-hydroxyflavanones and lycopene that inhibit cancer cell proliferation, tumor vascularization, and promotes normal cell differentiation.

Cancer of the Prostate

Prostate cancer is associated with increased age over fifty and excess testosterone, positive family history, associated BRCA 1 and 2 gene markers, and high PSA (prostate-specific antigen) levels. Advanced disease with poor outcomes is particularly linked to obesity in African-American males.

Prevention is associated with a reduction in dietary fat intake (red meat and dairy products) and an increased intake of cruciferous vegetables (broccoli, cauliflower, kale) with sulforaphane and indole glucosinolates that reduce risk of progression; pomegranate polyphenols with high antioxidant activity to inhibit proliferation, invasion and metastasis of cancer cells; Brazil nuts with selenium, vitamin E tocopherols; lycopene in cooked tomatoes; and catechins in green tea.

Natural Health of the Musculoskeletal System/ Bone Health

Osteoporosis is bone loss related to ageing due to the imbalance of more bone being lost than being formed. It is more pronounced in post-menopausal women due to decreased bone density mass with low levels of estrogen, which may lead to an increased incidence of hip, wrist, and vertebral fractures. There is a 50 percent risk of fractures in postmenopausal women, and 25 percent risk in men over the age of sixty. Women over the age of sixty-five should be tested routinely with a DEXA bone scan.

Prevention with the conventional medication, estradiol (Premarin) is effective in reducing menopausal symptoms and risk of osteoporosis. However, this is countered by the risk of ovarian, breast, and uterine cancers. A diet that includes soy and low-fat or non-fat dairy products, vitamin C and D, calcium, and magnesium is a natural way of preventing osteoporosis.

Foods that help prevent osteoporosis:

Soy (tofu, edamames, soymilk, miso, tempeh)	Vit. D (milk, eggs, non-fat dairy, sunshine)	Vit. C (citrus, acerola, rose hips, carambolas)	Dark leafy greens (broccoli, kale, collards)
Calcium fortified juices	Sardines, salmon	Black-eyed peas	black strap molasses

Poppy and sesame seeds	Almonds	Figs, bananas, apples	Yogurt
Mushrooms	Sweet potatoes	Grapes, raisins, wine	Peanut butter

Supplements that help prevent osteoporosis:

Calcium carbonate 1,200 mg/d	Calcium citrate 1,500 mg/d	Magnesium 200 to 400 mg/d
Soy 80 to 200 mg/d	Calcitrol (Vit D) 600 to 800 IU/d	Zinc, copper, boron, manganese

Avoid excess caffeine, colas, and salt as they increase calcium loss. High intake of vitamin A from retinol, fluoride, oxalates, phosphorus, and strontium may directly damage bone tissue. Vitamin A from fish oil, vegetables, and fruit and beta-carotene from carrots, spinach, cantaloupe, and tomatoes is good for bone health.

Botanicals to help prevent and treat osteoporosis include horsetail with high amounts of silica and available in the form of Osteosil, may improve bone density and works with calcium to improve general bone health. Red clover is a phytoestrogen which reduces bone loss especially in the lumbar spine.

Exercise with weights, strength training, and balance will improve bone health.

Fibromyalgia is total body pain involving muscles, nerves, bone, and joint stiffness, headaches, sudden fatigue, insomnia, and exaggerated pain response to pressure. The cause is purported to be due to an imbalance in the immune system between pro-inflammatory and anti-inflammatory cytokines, which affects nerve cells directly. Since it is often associated with other inflammatory conditions like obesity, arthritis, and anxiety/depression disorders, prevention and natural treatment are directed to control in these directions.

Prevention can be pursued through regular exercise and the release of natural endorphins with swimming, yoga, and cardio/aerobic fitness training and a diet high in organic fruit, vegetables, whole grains, extra virgin olive oil (antioxidants for DNA repair), omega 3 fish oils to improve the immune system and the avoidance of all processed foods and environmental toxins. Supplementation with magnesium 250 mg and calcium 500 mg daily is recommended. The botanicals, boswellia, turmeric, and ginger are excellent for reducing inflammation and cayenne peppers with capsaicin are effective in reducing nerve pain. Insomnia can be reduced or eliminated with melatonin 3 to 10 mg at bedtime, and energy and mood can be increased with relaxation techniques like breathing exercises, biofeedback, and cognitive behavior therapy. Massage improves blood flow to the muscles and nerves, and acupuncture improves meridian flow. Herbal teas with anamú and moringa have been beneficial in reducing inflammation.

Natural Health of the Brain and Nervous System

Stress, from emotional and/or physical factors, leads to the overproduction of cortisol by the hypothalamic-pituitary-adrenal system and epinephrine and norepinephrine by the adrenal glands, which puts the body into the fight (sympathetic) phase with a rise in heart rate, blood pressure, and blood sugar, anxiety, heartburn, and digestive system shutdown. Chronic stress leads to prolonged and periodic release of cortisol causing decreased appetite, weight loss, intermittent recurrent heart palpitations, a dysfunctional immune system leaving the body susceptible to disease, insomnia, and gradual long-term damage to organ systems. Conventional treatment of symptoms is not the answer.

Prevention is directed at removing or reducing the causes. Step 1: reduce the intake of caffeine and other stimulants like saturated fats, alcohol, and sugar which interfere with rest, relaxation, and sleep. Reduce anxiety promoting news, contact with others with agitated minds, and upsetting situations. Consider taking an anti-stress vitamin formula with vitamin C and E, calcium, potassium, B complex, zinc, and magnesium, which particularly reduces the stress response. Borage oil inhibits abnormal adrenalin release. Valerian root, calcium-magnesium citrate, chamomile, and St. John's wort have nerve-calming activity. Aromatherapy with lavender, energy medicine, homeopathy, massage, and breathing techniques may lower cortisol on the physical level, while prayer, meditation, laughter, and yoga work on the emotions. Bellows breathing is effective in situations of acute stress, while abdominal breathing works for chronic stress. The 4-7-8 breathing technique changes the hyper-fight or flight sympathetic system over to the calmer parasympathetic system. A diet rich in fruit, vegetables, and whole grains in multiple small meals offer balance and healing to the nervous system, while intense physical activity like walking or running at least thirty minutes a day, five days a week, can release calming endorphins and burn off excess adrenalin. Adaptogens like ashwagandha, rhodiola rosea, eleuthero root, schisandra, reischii mushrooms, and panax ginseng, are indicated for stress, emotional imbalance, lack of vitality and stamina, and to counteract fatigue and insomnia.

How we frame the matter and how we react to the stressor is of utmost importance. Coping mechanisms may help depending on the individual and the situation. All the best methods and solutions depend on five basic factors: physical and mental fitness, high-energy diet, strong social network, adequate rest (sleep), and a clear, calm mind.

Anxiety disorder is an excessive and persistent sense of apprehension caused by environmental and biological events that trigger high adrenalin release with large amounts of oxygen shifted to the brain and muscles resulting in sweating, palpitations, breathing difficulty and feelings of losing control to stress. The reaction is panic without apparent danger, dread, confusion, and impaired judgement and reasoning. Conventional treatment involves sedative and tranquilizer "pills" and various levels of cognitive behavioral and psychotherapy.

Prevention and control consist of knowing that the panic will not harm you. When symptoms arise, start the counteraction. Think positive, not negative, start the breathing four counts inhale; seven counts hold; and eight counts exhale through the mouth. Repeat four to five times to shift from sympathetic to parasympathetic system.

Especially for chronic anxiety, pursue a diet of omega 3 fatty acids (cold-water fish, walnuts, flaxseed), vitamin B6 and B12 for nerve health, vitamin C for antioxidant protection from DNA cellular damage. Botanicals indicated for anxiety control are chamomile, passionflower, clover blossom, green tea, hops (beer), valerian, and lemonbalm. Adjunctive therapies like hypnosis, autogenic biofeedback, guided imagery, acupuncture, acupressure, reikki sound and color therapy in energy medicine, and aromatherapy are all evidence-based effective.

Exercise regularly to burn off excess adrenalin and release endorphins and stabilize serotonin, the "feel good" hormone.

Depression disorder involves habitual thoughts of worthlessness, low self-esteem, and progressive isolation. The brain makes the chemical messenger hormone serotonin and dopamine from proteins, which determines the "quality "of emotions, thoughts, and reactions to stressful life events. The conventional treatment consists of a first line of antidepressants to keep serotonin levels high. Overdose or hypersensitivity could lead to confusion, tremors, lethargy, heart palpitations, seizures, suicidal thoughts, impulsive dangerous behavior, anxiety, and hallucinations. Cases of long-term use leading to addiction are well known. There is a physiological need to have serotonin and dopamine available for nerve endings, but too much is bad to worse.

Prevention takes the form of counselling in mind-body medicine by motivating self-esteem and healthy social connections in the teenage years. Know that since placebo studies, belief that the action of a medication will work, shows equivalence to antidepressants, the mind-body connection can cure the disorder. In depression, regular intense exercise is particularly effective. The release of endorphins, participation, toxin elimination, improved appearance, and improved brain blood flow and function appear to equal the response to antidepressants. Sustained exercise with endurance and improved flexibility, like walking, swimming, running, and gym workouts, is the most effective. Anti-obesity and elimination diets are recommended. Omega 3 fatty acids, with EPA (eicosapentanoic acid) 1,200mg, and DHA (docosahexaenoic acid) 900mg as cod liver oil and fish oil, improve cognition and mood, increase levels of natural brain neuro-steroids, and are essential for normal cell membrane function.

Botanicals like St. John's wort 300mg three times a day for three weeks at a time assists the brain in making serotonin, promotes calmness, and supports healthy sleep patterns. Valerian is a purely non-addictive herbal that inhibits the nerve impulses that prevent the body from having an uninterrupted sleep. Borage oil and gingko biloba are good for older people.

Care should be taken with massage and reiki as these involve "touching" and the sensitivity may not be good for depression. Hypnosis can reframe the situation and address it from different angles. Relaxation techniques like progressive muscle action and breathing techniques may physiologically instill a renewed feeling of well-being. Energy medicine addressing the Chakras, can redirect the blockage in depression, and relieve anger, grief and abuse. Acupuncture studies have shown success in re-directing the Qi to stimulate synthesis of norepinephrine and serotonin.

Neurodegenerative Disorders

Dementia is the term used for general abnormal memory loss associated with multiple brain blood vessel breakdown, alcoholism, trauma, and viral and genetic disease. Risk factors are advancing age over sixty-five, midlife obesity with high intake of dairy products, vascular disease, smoking, hypertension with high systolic blood pressure, diabetes, and reduced exercise, which lead to the formation of atherosclerotic plaques that rupture, clot, and cause blockage of arteries in the brain.

Prevention of general dementia and age-related memory loss (*periodic lapses with return to normal*), Coenzyme Q10, 100 to 500mg a day, coconut water/oil, and coffee daily reduced the risk and appeared to improve the symptoms. NSAIDS 200mg and aspirin 81mg (low dose) appeared to be protective to blood vessels of the brain. High intake of multiple antioxidants reduced the risk and time of onset and but did not stop the progression once established.

Alzheimer's is a form of dementia in which short-term memory, cognitive thinking, language and reasoning are affected by the formation of plaques and neurofibrillary tangles associated with recurrent injury from multiple mini-strokes, which leads to inflammation and further damage to the synapses and total loss of function. Defective white blood cells (microglia) of the immune system designated to protect the brain change and start to consume the amino acid, arginine, needed by the brain to function. The risk factors of genetics, age over sixty-five, toxin exposure, poor circulation and poor health, all contribute to causing these cells to change. A prominent factor not usually listed is the reduction or cessation of mental stimulation to which the individual was accustomed. The brain stops functioning at a high level.

Prevention is directed toward preservation of neuron health, through learning and memory exercise, and nutrients to promote healthy brain cells and active blood vessels. To remain *mentally active*, read, do crossword puzzles, play music, pursue ongoing education, travel, engage in hobbies, volunteer, and get involved with positive reinforcement. Above all, learn something new, a language, take an art class, ballroom dancing, computer class, writing, nature outings, or gardening. Keep the brain engaged and active.

Exercise: Regular physical activity up to five days a week seriously reduces oxidative stress, improves brain blood circulation, increases hormone release, and stimulates nerve growth factors to maintain attention and decision making ability. Walking thirty minutes a day, five days a week, is a good start. Interjecting swimming, an organized sport, and a gym workout are good ideas. Exercise alone can account for up to a 20 percent improvement in memory and nerve growth factors, and protects against diseases like type 2 diabetes, hypertension, and high cholesterol that affect heart and vascular health.

A diet high in antioxidants such as the following:

1. *Omega 3* , supplement 1,000mg daily or wild caught salmon, sardines, tuna, mackerel, herring, freshly ground flaxseed, walnuts, and extra virgin olive oil, such as the Mediterranean diet, is highly anti-inflammatory, with nominal caloric restriction and benefits far outweighing the risks.

2. *Vitamins C* (500mg) *and E* (400 IU) to lower the levels of toxic homocysteine and six servings fruit and dark leafy green vegetables daily to neutralize and reverse oxidative stress. Ingest a *multivitamin* daily with folic acid 800mcg and B vitamins (B6 20mg, B12 500mcg) for nerve health and repair.

3. *Detoxification* and regular elimination weekly, with lemon juice, apple cider vinegar, and olive oil.

4. *Turmeric* and *Ginger* daily with cayenne pepper spice added to meals two to three times a week to reduce inflammation.

5. *Aspirin* 81mg and/or *NSAIDS* 200 mg daily to improve blood flow. Beware of side effects on the liver and gastrointestinal system.

6. High intake of *arginine* rich foods, like nuts, seeds, coconut oil/water/meat, dark chocolate, oats, whole wheat, and gelatin. Be aware that arginine may trigger recurrent herpes cold sore lesions.

7. *Caffeine* stimulates the central nervous system and is good for Alzheimer's prevention. However, more than two cups of coffee a day may be toxic and potentially addictive.

Social connections must be sought, formed, and maintained. A strong circle of family and friends serve to stimulate cognitive function. If one is alone, join groups, church, community volunteer work, any organization that provides social contact.

Above all, *chronic stress* must be kept to a minimum. Physical and emotional factors that lead to anxiety and/or depression must be held in check with a positive attitude, strong social ties, and body and mind exercise.

Supplements for Dementia/Alzheimer's are available but whole foods are better. Gingko biloba, omega 3 (DHA) and EPA, ALA, GLA,_fish oils, vitamin C and E, flaxseed, evening primrose, and borage oil; avocado and coconut oil; Aswagandha, an antistress adaptogen; lemon balm and valerian tea for sedation; sage, rosemary, and thyme tea for circulation; turmeric and ginger for inflammation; moringa leaf, one teaspoon daily in cooking or as a tea, improves cognitive function and lowers risk. Brain foods like coconut, maca root, chocolate, macambo nuts, camu camu, and lucuma all have high protein and vitamin C content.

Avoid exposure to toxins and pollution, in the form of pesticides, insecticides, heavy metals, smoking, cooking in aluminum foil, and plastics. Do not drink water frozen in plastic bottles or store hot food in plastic containers. The BPA contained is toxic to nerve cells.

Prevent insomnia. Get good physiological no side effect rest with melatonin 3 to 10mg at bedtime. Try acupuncture, a relaxation massage, and mind-body balancing yoga to keep the systems toned and in tune.

Suggested Must-Do Daily for Prevention of Alzheimer's Disease

Dietary Antioxidants: Omega 3, coconut oil (cooking), coconut water, vitamin C, moringa, memory tea (rosemary, sage, thyme and ginkgo); + a multivitamin, + aspirin 81 mg.

Physical activity: walk, run, swim, visit the gym five days a week; twenty to thirty minutes each day.

Mental activity: daily puzzles, new languages, read, engage.

Social connection: volunteer, group, conversation, positive attitude; maintain, renew and form new relationships, globalize

Control Hypertension

(This is a strong factor for multiple-stroke dementia.)

Avoid smoking, excess alcohol, aluminum products, exposure to all neurotoxic pesticides, BPA and BPS plastics, and all heavy metals.

Parkinson's disease results from the loss of dopamine producing cells in substantia nigra region of the brain associated with exposure to environmental toxins (pesticides) that damage the cellular mitochondria, partial genetic impairment of detoxification pathways, and oxidative stress linked to excess iron deposits, leading to slow movements, stooped posture, and alternating tremors and rigidity.

Prevention may be directed to a diet high in antioxidants for their free radical scavenging and heavy metal chelating activity. Omega 3 with alpha lipoic acid (ALA), NADH (nicotinamide adenine dinucleotide) 5 to 10 mg, and Coenzyme Q10 200mg are known to protect the mitochondria from free radicals. Green and black tea with polyphenols and catechins, improve iron metabolism. Foods rich in isothiocyanates, like broccoli, kale, fava beans, and cabbage and coffee, two cups a day, can increase dopamine, the message-carrying brain chemical that is often deficient in Parkinson's.

There is a whole range of conventional medications from carbidopa-levodopa (Sinemet) and dopamine agonists like bromocriptine (Parlodel) and pergolide (Permax), plus amantadine (Symmetrel) and rorpinirole (Requip). Glitazone pills for diabetes, also helps to reduce the risk of Parkinson's, while also being linked to serious heart and bladder problems, as well as cancer in rats.

> Healthy people do not need nor take pharmaceutical drugs because they allow nature to keep them in balance. (A. L. Anduze, MD)

Epilepsy/Seizure disease consists of a sudden surge of abnormal electrical signals in the brain stimulated by excitotoxins, stressors/triggers like radiation, high-frequency sounds, energy efficient lights, microwave and video games and resulting in loss of consciousness or not, stiffness or rhythmic movements, abnormal sounds, confusion, and incontinence. Conventional treatment is with an arsenal of anticonvulsant drugs aimed at suppression (phenobarbital) and often with tremendous side effects like aplastic anemia and cancer.

Prevention entails a diet high in zinc, as its deficiency is strongly associated with seizures. Take lots of magnesium which may be in the form of pure grade Epsom salts (MgSO4), one-half teaspoon daily, magnesium supplements or whole food like almonds, cashews, peanuts, halibut fish, and dark leafy greens like spinach and kale. The botanicals, valerian and kava kava are anticonvulsant and antispasmodic. Skullcap and lobelia are calmative muscle relaxers. Epilepsy has been linked to Vitamin B1 (thiamine) deficiency, so adding this to diet should be of some help. Recently cannabadiol from cannabis sativa and indica has been shown to reduce the frequency of episodes, by occupying the CB1 and two brain receptors.

Avoid all bad food: white products like sugar, flour, rice, bread, salt, or processed food should not be in your pantry.

Insomnia is a sleep disorder where the inability to fall or stay asleep leaves one functionally impaired for most of the day. A sleep of either over eight hours and under five hours is not good for proper metabolism and function. The normal sleep should be between six to seven hours for the average adult. Narcolepsy, excessive daytime sleep with sudden muscle weakness and "frequent "sleep attacks;

restless legs syndrome (RLS) when aches and pains in the legs interfere with normal sleep, and sleep apnea, when gasping, snoring, and momentary intermittent suspensions of breathing interrupt the normal pattern, are all forms of sleep disorder.

Prevention is achieved by several basic tenets. Discontinue adverse sleep countering behavior like smoking, alcohol intake, noise, caffeine, and heavy fatty meal at bedtime. Leaving "worries" at the bedside by journaling and discarding the unpleasant information, doing light to moderate exercise followed by a warm bath with relaxing essential oils , guided imagery or music are all good support. Local remedies like chicken soup, graviola (soursop), chamomile, passionflower, and valerian teas all offer varying degrees of relaxation leading to a restful sleep. Lemon balm is FDA approved for sleep disorders. Instead of taking a chance with the deep sleep and side effects of "sleeping pills," melatonin 3 to 10 mg one hour before bedtime to regulate sleep rhythms, or 5-HTP (tryptophan) 100mg to raise serotonin levels that regulate sleep, are two good remedies, which though they have to be taken regularly for several days before effects are noted, are not habit forming and there are little or no side effects upon arising. Going to bed at the same time every night, on comfortable bedding, in a quiet dark relaxing environment is also contributory to a good night's sleep.

Autonomic Nervous System

Autism, ADD, ADHD with strong genetic/toxin related causes involve inflammation of the nerve and brain cells associated with exposure to chemicals, pollutants and heavy metals, refined sugars, and food additives, that lead to immune system deficiencies and nutritional imbalances from deficient essentials like calcium, magnesium, iodine, iron, and zinc; and excesses of copper, lead, mercury, cadmium, aluminum and nickel. Attention deficit disorder and attention deficit hyperactivity disorder occur mostly in young children who display characteristic symptoms of inappropriate crying, head banging, refusal of affection, hyperactivity, poor attention span, opposition to everything, poor coordination, aggression, inconsistent energy stores, and multiple allergies are countered by unusual multitasking, spontaneity and artistic creativity. Blood chemistry may reveal several vitamin and mineral deficiencies, and tendencies to hyper-allergenicity. Conventional treatments include psychostimulant medications like Ritalin, sedatives like Adderall for seven-year-olds, and selective norepinephrine receptor inhibitors like Strattera, together with the horrendous side effects of seizures, growth suppression, angina, blood pressure irregularities and concomitant depression. Natural treatments combine several different less intrusive approaches.

Prevention through nutrition involves the complete avoidance of refined sugars, all omega-6 pro-inflammatory foods those packaged with additives and synthetic chemicals, artificial flavorings and sweeteners like aspartame and MSG, all sodas and highly allergenic products like whole milk, candies, milk chocolate, cheese, and wheat. Instead, eat a balanced diet of good fats, low glycemic carbohydrates and plant-based protein, high in organic fresh fruit and vegetables devoid of pesticides. Take a multivitamin with zinc, iron and magnesium, vitamin B1, choline, and omega 3 (500 to 1000mg) daily to improve the growth of brain and nerve cell membranes. Reduce stress. Basic encounters should be devoid of yelling, lecturing, warnings, and bargaining. Positive reinforcement by applauding, laughter and the act of calming down, goes a long way. The routine use of low dose aspirin (81mg) to prevent abnormal clotting if indicated should be continued. Be aware that several foods, like garlic, ginger, ginkgo biloba, and fenugreek also exhibit blood thinning activity.

Botanicals like the bark of the French maritime pine tree give pycnogenol and polyphenols, which are potent antioxidants against nerve cell damaging free radicals, raise levels of glutathione and normalizes adrenaline to maintain a calm state. Valerian and lemon balm give a calming effect without the need of narcotics, and the ginseng 200mg/50mg ginkgo biloba combination is quite effective. Therapies like neurobiofeedback, guided imagery, hypnosis, yoga, and meditation can achieve significant behavior modification. Traditional Chinese medicine (TCM) offers acupuncture to restore the qi energy, homeopathy that is individualized, adequate sleep with assistance from melatonin, strenuous exercise in organized sports to increase endorphins and reduce cortisol, and urging of social connections to make and keep friends are all basics in the management of these relatively modern disorders.

Natural Health of the Cardiovascular System

Heart disease that leads to angina, congestive heart failure, arrhythmias, and myocardial infarction is associated with changes in blood composition leading to fatty plaque accumulation, thickening and hardening of arteries, and reduced blood flow, mostly associated with preventable problems, like lack of exercise, poor eating habits, overweight, and smoking. A small percentage is due to birth defects while the majority is linked to preventable conditions like high blood pressure, diabetes, excess alcohol, smoking, caffeine, and other drugs including medications. Risk factors include aging, male gender, positive family history, nicotine that constricts the blood vessels, carbon monoxide that damages the inner arterial lining, diet high in bad fats, salt, sugar and cholesterol, poor dental health and poor hygiene that lends to bacterial or viral infections.

Prevention through natural strategies include a low-fat, high-fiber balanced diet of whole grains, roughage (oats, brown rice, seeds, salad greens), fruit (apples, grapefruit, bananas, grapes, blueberries, cherries, lemon, oranges, and limes), cruciferous vegetables (broccoli, artichokes, cabbage, carrots, cauliflower), and good fats like nuts, seeds, olive oil, flaxseed, and wheat germ. A handful of nuts a day reduces heart disease by some 60 percent. Omega 3 fish oils to reduce the effects of atrial fibrillation and lots of garlic daily are extremely beneficial to heart health. Though one to two "drinks" a day for men and one for women has been promoted, one should be very careful about alcohol intake given the presence of risk factors. The botanicals, hawthorn berry (160 to 900mg daily) a cardiac regulator, and horse chestnut, an antioxidant for reducing varicosities are well known and proven. Supplements like Coenzyme Q10 (100 to 300mg daily), L-carnitine (3g daily), pycnogenol to lower the microalbumin level and a multivitamin with calcium, magnesium, copper, zinc, selenium, chromium and potassium, are good regulators to basic heart function. Vitamin C (500 to 1000mg daily) helps to reduce cardiac arrhythmias.

Exercise directed at aerobic capacity, decreases sensitivity to catecholamine drugs so that less may be needed, regulates heart rate and increases oxygen availability to the heart muscles. Acupuncture that redirects the flow of energy (Qi) can have a direct positive effect on the heart rhythm and biofeedback reduces the frequency and severity of palpitations through the awareness and perception to self-control of the arrhythmia. The relaxation response to breathing exercises, particularly the 4-7-8 technique that affects a change from the fight or flight anxiety laden sympathetic to the sit back and relax parasympathetic systems. Put the tip of your tongue at the roof of the mouth just between the two front teeth, exhale then and inhale to the count of 4, hold it to the count of 7, and exhale through the mouth to the count of 8. Repeat the sequence two to four times, with two to four sessions a day as needed. Yoga exercises with hatha body poses are helpful in breathing and balance.

Hypertension (high blood pressure) occurs when the small vessels become obstructed and the force against the blood vessel walls rises to an abnormal level. Arteries lose elasticity, constrict further, and the heart works harder, increasing the risk of stroke and complete breakdown, heart attack. Risk factors include aging; male gender; positive family history; being overweight; physically inactive; smoking; excess salt in the diet which causes water retention in the kidneys, that expands blood volume, and leads to increased pressure; deficiency of potassium, vitamin D and/ or a kidney enzyme deficiency; a high intake of alcohol with direct increase in pressure needed to metabolize it; high levels of stress; and certain chronic conditions like sleep apnea, kidney disease and diabetes.

Conventional treatment is to control the pressure ratio of blood out from the heart to blood into the heart, with pharmaceutical like ACE inhibitors, angiotensin receptor, calcium channel, and beta blockers, all effective but with unacceptable side effects.

Prevention and first line natural treatment is with a low fat, low salt diet to which whole grains and lots of fresh fruit and vegetables are added. Limit salt intake to one teaspoon a day. Avoid processed foods, excess caffeine, alcohol, and no smoking. Include omega 3 essential fatty acid foods, fish oil, good fats, and fiber like avocado, walnuts, chestnuts, mushrooms, fruits, and vegetables high in potassium like bananas, sweet potatoes, pomegranate, broccoli, kale, cantaloupe, figs, apricots, lemon, lime, and lots of garlic. Take a multivitamin with calcium, magnesium, folates, and vitamin C. Botanicals that help regulate blood pressure include cayenne pepper with tomato juice, green papaya, anamú, hibiscus, and juana la blanca tea. Most cardiovascular conditions respond well to acupuncture, hydrotherapy, hypnosis, tia chi, and yoga. Like the adverse effects of birth control pills, NSAIDS, diet pills, and decongestants, note that licorice root, guarana, kola nut, yerba mate, ginseng and yohimbe may cause variable and irregular blood pressure levels through vasodilation and constriction.

Exercise is a very important part of hypertension control and should include a good walk, a minimum of thirty minutes a day, three times a week with at least one good sweat to eliminate toxins and release the beneficial hormones.

Cholesterol ranges less than 200mg percentage for men and 220mg percentage for women may be a bit too rigid. These numbers assume that everyone has the similar body types and pursue similar degrees of physical activity. A discussion of individualization with your physician is suggested. An excess of low density lipoprotein (LDL) "bad" cholesterol may be made in the liver, released into the blood, contributes to the hardening of the arteries and formation of plaques on the inner walls, which lead to heart disease. "Good" cholesterol attaches to high density lipoproteins (HDL) and is carried away from the arteries back to the liver where is changed and made useful as hormones and beneficial fats. Excess cholesterol affects different individuals differently.

Prevention of accumulation of "bad" cholesterol is directed toward the diet that is low in saturated fat (animal protein, dairy, whole milk, cheese, butter, and red meat), no trans fats (junk food, snacks in bags, chips, crackers, and commercially baked cookies). Absolutely no smoking as it may directly lower levels of protective HDL cholesterol as well as release toxins that promote LDL oxidation leading to inflammation and raised levels of total cholesterol, triglycerides and breakdown of lipid metabolism. Eat plant-based antioxidant-laden proteins like one cup of nuts (walnuts, hazelnuts, almonds, cashews, pistachios) daily; bananas with potassium prevents plaque from sticking to vessel walls; natural cholesterol reducers like quinoa one-half cup has 90mg of magnesium; fiber rich oats, whole grains, cereals and wheat germ; legumes, beans, lentils, citrus, peas, carrots; good fats like olive oil, fish oils, skinless chicken; cinnamon one-half teaspoon a day that reduces cholesterol by 30 percent plain yogurt that provides probiotics for proper digestion and absorption; red wine and dark chocolate with antioxidant flavonoids, resveratrol and polyphenols. Botanicals like ginger, ginseng and green tea, vitamin B3 (niacin), Coenzyme Q10, Shiitake mushrooms, flaxseeds, guggol 1000mg three times a day, kutaki 100mg daily and red yeast rice 1200mg twice daily have all been shown to reduce cholesterol as compared to stains but with a minimum of side effects. The potential and possibility of transferring from statins to natural cholesterol control should be presented and discussed with your doctor, particularly if the side effects are debilitating and/or the levels are below the 200 to 220mg percent range.

Detoxification with a mixture of one teaspoon each of apple cider vinegar, lemon juice, and olive oil is an effective safe weekly cleanse.

Exercise to maintain ideal body weight (BMI in range of 18 to 22.4).

Circulation is affected by the same risk factors that affect blood and cardiovascular systems. A weak heart, plaques in the arteries, and veins with weak valves and poor tone, are the main causes of poor perfusion to organs and tissues, giving symptoms of easy and frequent fatigue, poor concentration and pedal edema.

Prevention and natural treatments are highlighted by blood pressure and cholesterol control. Increased hydration (drinking more water) is the hallmark of the dietary intake regimen. Limiting caffeine and alcohol to two a day or less, increasing protein fiber intake, like buckwheat and papaya products with antioxidants to improve blood flow, and supplementing with vitamins K and B complex to reduce platelet aggregation (clotting) and increase prostacyclin production to keep red blood cells "slippery" is also effective. Removal of heavy metal toxic deposits with chelation and fibrinolysis to dissolve existing blood clots by delivery of nitric oxide to the arterial endothelium are effective is done in the early stages. Botanicals to improve small blood vessel flow include geranium, ginkgo biloba, ginger, rosemary, sweet woodruff, cayenne and garlic.

Physically applying warmth/heat to the body parts with a hot water bottle or pack, and/or extra warm socks, will stimulate dilation of blood vessels and improve circulation.

Exercise by walking or other sustained movement will increase blood flow. Basic warm up stretches, yoga and tai chi are also effective. Effective manipulations include acupuncture, massage, and hydrotherapy.

Stroke or cerebrovascular accident is caused by poor or blocked blood flow to the brain resulting in localized cell death usually manifested as the inability to move or feel one side of the body, decreased speech or comprehension, and decreased vision on one side. Anticoagulants are the standard of care but must be administered within minutes in the acute phase if they are to be effective. Risk factors that are preventable and treatable, include drug abuse (especially cocaine, amphetamines, and alcohol), smoking, atrial fibrillation, hypertension, diabetes, high cholesterol, sickle-cell disease, and positive history of heart disease. Identifiable and incurable factors include age, the most important, family history, and genetic heart disease.

Conventional treatment with anticoagulants, blood thinners, coumarin, and warfarin-like medications, thrombin inhibitors, like aspirin, statins, Plavix, Pradaxa, eliquil, and others is also accompanied with side effects. Spontaneous hemorrhage and persistent bleeding occur often and are difficult to reverse or control. It is definitely more practical and plainly more sensible to address and correct the risk factors than to suffer the effects of post incident treatment.

Prevention is directed at blood pressure, blood sugar, and cholesterol control; stress reduction, smoking cessation, salt intake reduction, weight control, and no junk or processed foods. Implement an antioxidant-rich, low0fat diet with fruit and vegetables, especially with the blue and purple berries and red grapes (anthrocyanidins), omega 3 fish oils, flaxseed, and walnuts for inflammation reduction, and potassium-rich foods like lima and kidney beans, lentils, yogurt, and prunes. Botanicals that are antioxidants and active blood thinners (without the side effects) are garlic, ginger, ginkgo biloba, green tea, ginseng, gojiberry, feverfew, chamomile, boswellia, sage, St. John's wort, and dong quai. Cayenne pepper in large amounts has been shown effective in reducing inflammation and improving circulation.

In an otherwise healthy individual, aspirin, and statins are not recommended as prevention measures in light of the risks of adverse side effects.

Exercise regular, structured, and definitive is beneficial, as are yoga, tai chi, and other movement and balance arts.

Blood

Anemia is a group of disorders of the blood in which there is a reduction in the number of red blood cells and/or amount of hemoglobin molecules available to bind and carry oxygen to the tissues. Iron deficiency anemia results from low levels of iron, pernicious anemia from low vitamin B12 or B6 and in folic acid anemia (another B vitamin type), there is a reduced production of red blood cells. The risk factors include excessive loss of blood during menstruation, injury, peptic ulcer, colon cancer, and long term aspirin use with internal bleeding.

Prevention is with increased intake of iron rich foods, like red meat, liver, egg yolks, cereals, fortified raisins, fish, poultry, legumes, whole grain bread, green leafy vegetables, dried apricots, prunes, and soy beans. If supplemental iron with folic acid is taken, make sure to include vitamin C to help with basic absorption and dietary fiber should be increased to prevent constipation. Botanicals include those high in iron, folates, and B vitamins, like dandelion, goji juice, noni tea, milk thistle, artichoke, anise, caraway seeds, vervain, blue-green algae (spirulina), burdock, and comfrey.

Natural Health of the Respiratory System

One may promote lung health by improving air quality with indoor plants like areca palms, mother-in-law tongue, ferns, and rhododendrons, which provide clean oxygen and absorb many pollutants.

Asthma is a condition in which the airways become inflamed, swell, and produce extra mucus leading to a narrowing of the air passages of the lungs. Triggers like cold air, exercise, and external allergens are usually associated with reactions (allergy) where hypersensitive immune cells act with hyperactive lung cells to cause shortness of breath, wheezing, chest tightness, and difficulty breathing. Conventional treatments include immediate application of corticosteroids to suppress the immune response and bronchodilators to open constricted respiratory smooth muscles. Use of and inhaler should be no more than one to two puffs a day.

Prevention and natural treatment is aimed at diet change to reduce the "allergens" by eliminating wheat, corn, and dairy products and taking in omega 3 fish oils, fruits, vegetables, legumes and walnuts with anti-inflammation properties. Brazil nuts with selenium that is highly protective of asthma, vitamin C, six ounces daily and vitamin E foods like spinach, quinoa, kale, and almonds are recommended. Botanicals like Muang (ephedra tea), tylophora, and lobelia can break an acute attack through bronchodilation. Black tea with theophylline, whole licorice, with its steroid-like response without the side effects, peppermint and eucalyptus to relax bronchioles are effective long term. Stinging nettle and quercetin capsules, and Echinacea in high doses (6 to 9 grams) are good for acute reactions.

Exercise to mobilize the fluids and increase blood flow is beneficial. Breathing exercise like slow balloon breathing and other relaxation techniques can improve the lung efficiency. Reduction of stress related incidents and relief with fenugreek, B complex vitamins, and regular use of an adaptogen (tonic) like ashwagandha, can provide stability and reduction in frequency of attacks.

Emphysema is a type of chronic obstructive pulmonary disease (COPD), in which damage to the walls of the small air sacs in the lung result in the collapse of the airways and permanent obstruction of air flow into the lungs.

Bronchitis is the inflammation of the bronchiole tubes that carry air to and from the lungs. The reduced lung capacity is manifested as repeated bouts of shortness of breath, chronic cough, weight loss, fatigue and "barrel chest." Risk factors include age between forty to sixty, cigarette smoking and exposure to second-hand smoke that directly damage lung tissue, occupational exposure to air pollutants like chemical fumes and dust, heating fuel, car exhaust, and presence of bronchial asthma. Conventional treatments include regular use of bronchodilators like albuterol, atrovent, and ventolin, and often overuse of antibiotics which are prone to bacterial resistance, steroids, with side effects of weakened bones, diabetes and hypertension, and supplemental oxygen.

Prevention includes mandatory immediate cessation of smoking and avoidance of exposure to all pollutants. Theophylline in teas is very effective for its anti-inflammation and bronchodilation activities. Coenzyme Q10 at 60mg taken twice daily with meals appears to improve oxygen absorption and use in the lungs, Cordyceps capsules (a medical mushroom) improves lung efficiency and slows the progression of lung disease, and N-acetyl cysteine (NAC) decreases phlegm and thins excess mucus.

Sleep apnea is the term given to a disorder in which breathing repeatedly stops and starts, leading to various degrees of oxygen deprivation during sleep. There are two types, obstructive, resulting in blockage of the airway by soft tissues of the throat that relax and collapse and central, resulting when the brain fails to signal muscles to breathe, like in stroke and neuromuscular diseases. Risk factors include being male, over age forty, overweight with a large neck (greater than seventeen inches) large nostrils and tongue, associated snoring, GERD, nasal septum deviation, allergies, and sinusitis.

Prevention is by changing position, raise chin up and forward, sleep on side, extra pillows, weight loss, blood pressure control, devices to keep airways open, and a strict avoidance of nighttime alcohol, smoking and sleeping pills up to four hours before sleep. Hot tea with chamomile and 1 teaspoon of olive oil has been purported to help.

Natural Health of the Metabolic/ Endocrine Systems

Diabetes type 1 is associated with genetic congenital absence of insulin making capacity; type 2 is adult onset, insulin resistance/low insulin capacity; "type 3" is associated with overeating, inactivity, and obesity. Once on insulin, always required as the cells that make even a little insulin shut down and cease to function. Once on oral hypoglycemic, one may reduce the dosage by adding natural treatments, exercise, and weight control. Persistent high blood sugar affects and damages every organ system and tissue type, progressing lower limb amputations, blindness from retinopathy, kidney failure, and heart failure.

Prevention and natural treatment are best achieved through a combination of exercise and adherence to strict dietary rules. Exercise loses fat and lowers blood sugar improves health of cells and changes them from insulin resistant to insulin sensitive. Physically active muscles can extract glucose from the blood better than sedentary muscles. A poor circulation from lack of exercise results in reduced oxygen to cells and allows a poor diet to destroy health. Too much "fat" in the blood stream blocks the effectiveness of insulin. Minimum regimen consists of three (3) times a week, walk, run, swim, gym, that breaks a sweat (elimination of toxins). Being overweight is often associated with inflammation, which is associated with diabetes through the disruption of cells that function in insulin pathways.

A diet high in fruit and vegetables (50 to 60 percent), low in good quality protein (10 to 15 percent), and moderate in good quality mono and polyunsaturated fats (30 to 40 percent) will deliver enough energy and nutrition without having to rely on low quality carbohydrates. A diabetic *can* eat healthy fruit like papaya, grapefruit, oranges, apple with pectin fiber and berries; *can* eat vegetables like spinach, broccoli, lentils, pumpkin, asparagus, chayote squash, onions, garlic, avocados, and cucumber, all magnesium-rich foods; *can* eat beans, lean meats, poultry, whole grains, omega-3 fish, walnuts, and freshly ground flaxseed. The problem lies in the *amount* of food ingested. The energy intake must equal the energy expended. They must balance. Maintain normal weight, eat small frequent meals, reduce starches, eat only low glycemic sugars, and watch portion size of each one.

Avoid high glycemic sugars, all sodas and sweetened drinks, no saturated or trans-fats, no packaged foods, sugary cereals, commercially prepared cookies. Peas, potatoes, and corn are high carbohydrates, while spinach, carrots, cucumbers, and mushrooms are low.

Supplement with soy, which has genistein to reduce early retinopathy; garlic with allicin to reduce inflammation and deliver a host of healthy phytochemicals; coffee is actually good for type 2 diabetes as the caffeine improves insulin sensitivity; Chromium 1000mg a day helps with blood sugar regulation; and Alpha lipoic acid 100mg daily is an antioxidant that enhances glucose uptake and inhibits sugar attachment to protein.

Botanicals that have been shown to help reduce blood sugar are cinnamon extract, gymnema sylvestre, fenugreek seed, aloe vera, lemon tea, Chaya leaves, and psyllium.

Remember the three most important ways for blood sugar control: diet, exercise, and medications.

Low Glycemic Foods (Good)

skim or low fat milk	plain yogurt	soy (tofu, miso, soymilk)
apple, plum, orange	sweet potato (yam)	oat bran bread
oatmeal	brown rice, quinoa, basmati	pasta (al diente)
lentils, kidney beans	Chick peas	carrots, spinach, kale

Obesity is identified as body weight relative to height, over the BMI (body mass index) of 30, due mainly to excess fat. Normal body weight index is 22 t 24.9. The principal cause is more calories in than out and has little or nothing to do with eating fatty foods, as "low-fat" and "no fat" foods also have calories, plus added sugar (carbohydrates) and chemicals. Risk factors include genetic body type, family history; culture where overeating is traditional; not paying attention to good nutrition by eating what pleases, not what is nutritional; high-calorie junk food (appetizers, breadsticks, chips, packaged sweets and fried products); regular and diet sodas (sugar and synthetic sweeteners trigger increased appetite, eat more so that one to two drinks a day result in added calories); sedentary "TV snacking" increases caloric intake while decreasing caloric burn; not enough or too much sleep resulting in disrupted metabolism; "combo meals" eating more than you need; skipping meals then going into prime fat-storage mode and overeating at the next opportunity; buffet style eating; binge and emotional upset eating; poor diet, bad food, with high fat, high carbohydrate content; metabolic dysfunction (pituitary, adrenals, thyroid); associated medications (Paxil, Zyprexa, Thorazine, Allegra, and Prednisone). Obesity is associated with every disorder of the body and mind that is linked to chronic inflammation. A BMI that is 10 percent over normal (26) is overweight; 20 percent over normal (30) is obese and BMI of 40 or one hundred pounds pounds over normal is morbid obesity. Conventional treatments are with potent stimulants that raise the metabolic rates with concomitant increases in heart rate, pulse, blood pressure, palpitations, anxiety, and possible death, and diuretics which may result in serious potassium loss, which affects all organ systems but particularly the cardiovascular.

Prevention is most sanely directed at changes in dietary patterns. Four small meals a day; reducing the intake of carbohydrates to less than 40 percent of the meal, or reducing fat intake to 30 percent or less, leads to the most loss of weight in pounds. An increase in fiber and plant-based proteins to round out the diet; limit or cessation of all unhealthy food; decrease in portion size of each item to the amount that can fit into the palm of the hand; all help to lose weight. Evidence strongly supports the benefits of taking antioxidants foods with zinc, alpha lipoic acid, carnitine, cinnamon, green tea, Vitamin C and Vitamin E and is slightly weaker for omega-3, polyunsaturated fatty acids, Coenzyme Q10, green coffee beans, resveratrol, and lycopene for weight control. Drinking lots of water (eight to ten glasses a day) works as an effective appetite suppressant, as a catalyst in digestion and may burn up to three hundred calories of fat per day, and avoid constipation and bloating. Eating the good foods listed in table 1 in chapter 2, and strictly avoiding the bad foods in table 2, will strongly favor the maintenance of normal weight.

Taking medications do not and cannot address dysfunctional behavior patterns.

Physical activity must be increased and maintained concomitantly with changes in food choices, in order to get adequate weight reduction results. Deliberate, structured exercise consisting of thirty minutes minimum (walk, run, swim, gym) is crucial to effective weight loss. (Some 95 percent of participants will regain the weight in the absence of exercise). Exercise in the morning burns fat, in the afternoon, burns calories. A slow, long walk of forty-five to sixty minutes, five days a week, burns fat as well as tones and adds muscle.

Reduction of stress by improving sleep, biofeedback methods, and acupuncture greatly assists with weight loss. Supplementation with a complete multivitamin, with selenium and chromium, blood sugar regulators; green tea with fat-burning catechins; garlic to lower cholesterol; and choline and inositol to help with appetite suppression, blood sugar levels, and fat metabolism. Botanicals like flaxseed oil, kola nut, and ginger burn fat. Fruit like garcinia cambogia and hoodia gorgoni contain natural fat-burning hydroxycitric acid. Brewer's yeast and dandelion reduce food cravings; licorice and ginseng reduce cravings for sweets; red raspberry reduces appetite; and red clover clears appetite stimulating toxins.

Education on the basics of a good diet and nutrition with an optimum diet in which balance and regulation of bodily functions are the goals, can greatly contribute to weight management success.

Basic Rules for Weight Control

1. Attitude: prepare and enjoy a meal, preferably in good company,

2. Multiple small meals daily: four (breakfast, mid-morning, early afternoon, dinner).

3. Portion size: only amount of one food item that fits in the palm of your hand.

4. Balanced diet: equal amounts of protein and fats, more vegetables and fruit (carbs).

5. Fat-burning foods: cayenne pepper, cinnamon, green tea, omega-3 fish oils, fiber.

6. Drink water first thing in morning, in between and with every meal, at night; nine glasses daily.

7. Avoid all bad foods: trans fats, artificial sweeteners, fat substitutes, MSG, aspartame, processed

8. Digestion: add probiotics (yogurt), antacids (Tums), chamomile tea at night.

9. Elimination: high natural fiber, exercise (sweat), psyllium, flaxseed.

10. Exercise: burn fat in the morning, burn calories in the afternoon.

11. Botanicals: hoodia (tamarind), garcinia cambogia, raspberry leaf tea, green tea.

12. Sleep, stress reduction, relaxation exercises to reduce anxiety (do not eat).

Visualize your body as you want it to be.

Thyroid dysfunction can be high, overactive associated with unexplained changes in weight, appearance of goiter, eye signs of Graves disease, bulging eyes due to lid retraction, depression, sexual dysfunction, extreme fatigue, or low, underactive related to overweight, hair memory loss, cold tired, with brittle nails, and pedal edema. Risk factors include female gender, over age fifty, positive family history, pregnancy and post-partum period, cigarette smoking, overuse or deficiency of iodine, autoimmune diseases, and immunosuppressant, antiretroviral, antibody, lithium, amiodarone medications. Overeating or sensitivity to some foods is associated with thyroid goiter formation, like cabbage, broccoli, radishes, turnips, millet, kale, and Brussels sprouts.

Prevention is directed at maintaining a healthy functional thyroid gland. Eating wheatgrass, seaweed (kelp, spirulina, dulse, nuri), shellfish, saltwater fish, low-fat cheese, and ice cream with natural iodine will help to boost the thyroid function. Supplements like guggul 1,000mg daily help to regulate thyroid by reducing cholesterol levels. Ginseng and thyme tea daily will help to regulate blood circulation, an important thyroid function. Lemon balm is effective in balancing thyroid hormones.

Chronic fatigue syndrome may occur in the absence of obvious medical conditions. The diagnosis is suggested if one has four or more of the following symptoms: decreased short-term memory, low-grade fever, sire throat, tender lymph nodes, muscle pain, multi-joint pain without swelling or redness, headaches, restless sleep, and post-exercise malaise. These are signals of an immune system breakdown. Low energy levels can be related to deficiencies in vitamins and minerals and may also be associated with thyroid dysfunction.

Prevention and natural treatment to rebuild or enhance the immune system is primarily with magnesium/calcium combination and vitamin C supplement and whole foods. Adaptogens, tonics with rejuvenating activity, like eleuthero root for increasing mental activity and physical endurance; coenzyme Q10 for cellular energy production; ashwagandha, an antistress botanical to counteract fatigue and assist with better sleep; cordyceps, a mushroom that boosts energy and reduces high blood pressure; and panax ginseng, to boost immune system and add vitality. Any one or two of these together with moderate aerobic exercise and sensible nutrition, should produce beneficial results. Foods with B complex vitamins and iron, like fruit (apples, plums, berries), dark leafy green vegetables, whole grains, lean protein and plant-based fat (avocado) are needed to boost energy levels. Iron rich foods like beans, lentils, spinach, seeds, should be taken with vitamin C rich fruit to assist absorption. Supplementation with additional vitamin B12 may help to increase red blood cell formation and oxygen carrying capacity to cells. Be careful with energy bars as they sometimes contain an inordinate amount of sugar.

Digestive/Gastrointenstinal

Digestive tips, GI Health Promotion: Prevention

More than half of disease conditions are associated with "gut issues." Poor or incomplete absorption and assimilation of nutrients leaves the tissues and organs bereft and prone to malfunction. Newborns (fetuses) are born deficient in enzymes and catalysts necessary to breakdown and incorporate nutritious products properly. They are often given artificial food and a slew of antibiotics in the newborn period which totally renders their immune system nonfunctional. This is followed by GMO food without the proper markers, enzymes, catalysts, vitamins, and minerals, and then processed foods with toxins and damaged proteins, and expected to develop with proper digestion and elimination processes. Even as these deficiencies have clearly been identified and elucidated, the food and pharmaceutical industries hold sway on what is ingested and what is omitted often based on availability, affordability and awareness. Presently our "gut issues" include celiac disease and a large group of gluten-intolerant individuals, food allergies, gastroesophageal reflux disease (GERD), early gastrointestinal cancers, liver and gallbladder disorders, irritable bowel syndrome (IBS), and enteritis. Poor or faulty absorption of necessary nutrients is also linked to asthma, autism, diabetes, Alzheimer's, multiple sclerosis, Parkinson's, and other CNS disorders, liver, gallbladder, pancreas and spleen disorders, and arthritis.

Conventional treatment with strong antacids (Prilosec, Prevacid, Zantac) tend to reduce and inhibit normal enzyme production in the stomach while mainly treating symptoms. They ignore the "underlying cause," which can be bad food, poor eating habits, bad digestion, overuse of antibiotics and steroids and other products, which may interfere with absorption and lead ultimately to poor immune system function. The imbalance of bad to good bacteria results in poor digestion and in turn leads to bad digestion.

Prevention of digestive disorders begins with and is based upon good eating habits, which in turn results in the development and maintenance of good absorption mechanisms.

1. Eat in seated position, quiet, pleasant, and without distraction.

2. Eat the main meal at midday for good hydrochloric acid (HCL) release and utilization.

3. Eat slowly, chew well (X30 count with each mouthful).

4. Eat proteins first, salads last as heavier food needs fresher, stronger digestive juices.

5. Include a variety of foods, organic when possible, balanced diet.

6. Eat 75 percent steamed or raw food at least once daily.

7. Avoid ice cold or overly hot foods (oven or stove heated).

8. Use more red pepper (cayenne), reduces inflammation of the mucosa (less black pepper).

9. Use natural sea salt, extra virgin olive oil, cold pressed seed oil, or bee pollen (protein) with at least one meal daily.

10. Avoid drinking any beverages with meals (interferes with digestive juices).

11. Drink water after the meal to boost digestion.

12. Mild exercise after the meal boosts metabolism, which boosts digestion.

The composition of the diet should be foods with adequate digestive enzymes like protease, lipase, and amylase, which help with the digestion of proteins, fats, and carbohydrates, to break down food into smaller more absorbable entities. Adding bromelain from pineapples and papain from papaya is also a big help. Eat lots of fiber from fruit, raw vegetables, nuts, seeds, legumes, whole grains, and Brewer's yeast. Do not hesitate to use *probiotics* to replace bad with good bacteria. It is easy, it is inexpensive, and it works. Though in some cases they can counteract the indigestion related to gluten and lactose intolerance, preventing digestive issues is much easier than dealing with crises. Day-to-day stress, tension, poor eating habits, travel, exposure to toxins, and overuse of antibiotics may lead to a depletion of good bacteria. Probiotics, found in foods like yogurt, kefir, miso soup, and kimchi, are a replacement of good bacteria which help to digest food and synthesize nutrients like vitamins K, B complex, and certain essential fatty acids. It must be fresh, fermented, unpasteurized, and consist of a minimum of one billion live organisms. Note that pasteurization kills both harmful and beneficial organisms to the human body. The good bacteria eliminate the disease-causing bacteria in addition to stimulating and enlisting the immune system response. A daily dose of probiotics is especially indicated during periods of travel when and where the food content may be alien to the digestive tract as well as with antibiotic induced diarrhea. Supplements with *Lactobacillus rhamnosus* and /or *Saccharomyces boulari* are highly recommended two days before and daily during travel. In cases of weakened immunity or on immunosuppressive drugs, taking Lactobacillus rhamnosus, L. plantarum and L. salvarius, Bifidobacterium bifidum will help.

Enzyme-Rich Foods for Digestion

Seeds	Pineapple	Papaya	Kiwi	Aloe vera
Cabbage	Beets	Broccoli	Alfalfa sprouts	Celery
Arugula	Kefir (probiotic)	Kombucha	Shiitakemushroom	Kale

Chewing all food thoroughly adds saliva that is rich in digestive enzymes.

Avoid all artificially flavored food with chemicals, dyes, (aspartame, MSG, sucralose, diet sweeteners), highly processed oils, white flour, white sugar, white rice, white bread.

Be aware that gluten-free foods may not be what they seem. They may consist of sugary additives, processed fillers, nutrient-empty taste-good ingredients, starches and inflammatory oils. Only those with diagnosed celiac disease, and /or gluten allergy or sensitivity should pursue a gluten-free diet.

Detoxification of the gastrointestinal tract with two tablespoons (one ounce) each of lemon, olive oil, and apple cider vinegar once a week is a good basic regimen.

Eat Natural, Eat Organic, Eat Local

Gastroesophageal Reflux (GERD) is basic indigestion usually following a heavy fatty meal, characterized by irritation of the upper stomach and lower esophageal lining from backflow of excess bile fluids. Resulting in bloating, urgency to vomit, and difficult breathing, it is associated with an interaction of factors which include environmental, emotional, physiological, and cognitive behavioral stress.

Conventional treatments include antacids like Mylanta and Tums, some with narcotics, proton pump inhibitors like Prevacid and Prilosec, and H-2 blockers, like Tagamet and Pepcid, all of which reduce acid in the stomach.

Prevention consists of basic precautions like wearing loose clothing to reduce external pressure and eating at least two hours before bedtime so that adequate digestion can take place. Raising the head of the bed to almost sitting position and using relaxation techniques are also helpful. Keeping a diary of what affects you adversely and what does not; increasing fiber in the diet; staying hydrated; avoiding stimulants like caffeine and alcohol at night; aspirin, NSAIDS, birth control pills all irritate the stomach lining; avoid dairy products with slow digestion properties; and take green tea in daytime and chamomile tea at bedtime. Supplementing with deglycyrrhizinated licorice (DGL), two tablets or two tablespoons powder in warm water at bedtime or a teaspoon of powder between meals or chewable tablets as needed; 1,000mg of d-limonene every other day for three weeks; marshmallow root in between meals soothes inflamed intestines; slippery elm and Irish moss heal intestinal tissues; probiotics with meals help to stabilize the entire digestive tract, promote absorption, reduce LDL cholesterol, enhance bowel function and protect against toxins. Magnesium citrate (milk of magnesia) is a good old-fashioned regulator of digestion. A teaspoon of apple cider vinegar and honey and/or sarsaparilla with panax ginseng are good digestive tonics. Other stomach herbals include angelica, balmony, black elder, wild cherry, wormwood (artemesia), rhubarb, and raspberry leaf tea. Other good supplements are iberogast and sucralfate.

Gastritis is the inflammation and irritation of the stomach lining (mucosa) characterized by fullness after eating, indigestion, burning, abdominal pain, loss of appetite, and dark stools. The causes include infection by Helicobacter pylori bacteria, vitamin B12 deficiency, overuse of pain medications like aspirin and ibuprofen, and overuse of acidic or spicy food and drinks. Risk factors include excess alcohol intake, Crohn's disease (enteritis), HIV/AIDS, parasitic infections, and other viral and fungal infections. Stress is a major contributor. Prolonged and repeated bouts of gastritis may lead to peptic ulcers.

Conventional treatments with antacids that neutralize reactive stomach acids only relieve the symptoms.

Prevention begins with adopting good eating and digestive practices. In addition, there are several excellent natural products that reduce digestive tract inflammation, prevent ulcers, and cancer. Ginger tea, powder, and lozenges have proven gastro-protective activity and antioxidant scavenging repair. Chamomile tea has apigenin, which directly inhibits Helicobacter pylori bacteria and protects against cancer. Peppermint has anti-inflammation, antibacterial, and antispasmodic properties that reduce stomach lining inflammation. Strawberries reduce alcohol damage to the stomach lining by fermentation and absorption. Basil is effective against H. pylori as well. Fennel seeds, anise, and licorice relax the stomach muscles, and reduce inflammation and the risk of ulcers. Potato juice is alkaline and helps to neutralize excess stomach acid and promotes healing of a damaged lining.

Irritable bowel syndrome (IBS) is inflammation of the large intestine (colon) without tissue changes and is related to the overgrowth of pathogenic (bad) bacteria due to poor diet, toxins abuse, and stress. The resultant bloating (fullness after meals), cramps, diarrhea, constipation, and pain are due to excess gas produced by the bacteria and indicates that digestion is not functioning properly. Poor digestion is associated with arthritis, allergies, autoimmune diseases, and mood disorders due to the disruption of the immune system.

Prevention is directed at digestive health, dietary changes, and reduction of stress by natural means and without drugs. High quality probiotics, like VSL3 and S. boulardii, daily can re-balance the gut-immune system to digest food particles properly. Fruit with digestive enzymes should be added to help break down food particles while the gut heals. A zinc supplement is recommended to replace minerals lost to diarrhea. A high fiber diet to promote healthy bacteria, fish oil to reduce gut inflammation and a multivitamin to balance hormones and support assimilation of food, should restore a healthy digestive system. *Avoid* high sugar, alcohol, overuse of antibiotics, aspirin, and NSAIDS.

Enteritis/Crohn's disease is inflammation of the large intestine with tissue damage and possibility of associated cancer. An imbalance of the gut bacteria and poorly functioning enzymes due to overuse of antibiotics is a major cause. A weak or faulty immune system is also implied. It is often associated with celiac disease (gluten intolerance), which may be genetic or acquired.

Prevention and natural treatment are directed at rebuilding the immune system. The addition of probiotics with good bacteria to the diet is the main natural solution. Avoid gluten foods (until gut is in good enough condition to absorb and assimilate them). Civilization was built on wheat. How ironic it is that now so many people are wheat intolerant. Staple foods like rye, barley, hops (beer), pasta, flour, cereals, and oats, have been replaced with artificial foods like canned soups, lunch meats, hot dogs, salad dressings, GMO soy sauce, seasoned rice, and many others with additives. Touted as being gluten-free, just how healthy are they? If absolutely necessary, look for organic fruit, vegetables, beans, dairy, nuts, quinoa, and wild rice, which are gluten-free. Prebiotics, non-digestible carbohydrates like artichokes, honey, whole grains, bananas, onions, and garlic, provide nutrients for the probiotic bacteria, and fish oil for its anti-inflammation properties, are all recommended. Acupuncture releases endorphins (chemicals that block pain and strengthen the immune system, biofeedback relaxation therapy that self-monitors blood pressure body temperature, perspiration levels, blood flow, and brain waves, can help improve digestive function. Aloe vera juice, slippery elm bark, chamomile, and peppermint teas are all effective in soothing and calming the digestive tract tissues.

Cholecystitis is inflammation of the gallbladder due to irritation resulting from changes in the chemical constituents of the stored bile fluids and an accumulation of cholesterol and bile salts forming gallstones, or tumor formation leading to blockage of the bile duct. If not relieved, a rupture may lead to life-threatening circumstances. Risk factors include female gender, over age sixty, overweight, a diet high in fried foods, high fat and high cholesterol, pregnancy, diabetes, statin and estrogen medications, and poor digestive health.

Prevention lies in maintaining healthy normal weight, eating regular, well-balanced meals with some good fats that cause the gallbladder to empty on a regular basis. Foods with calcium (milk, leafy green vegetables) and low cholesterol content are preferred.

Pancreatitis is the inflammation of the pancreas, which affects the normal production of digestive enzymes which break down nutrients like fats and proteins, as well as hormones, like insulin and glucagon, needed for sugar metabolism. The abnormal function may result in self-digestion of the gland itself through autoimmune processes. The main mechanism involves gall stones that migrate through the bile duct and block the pancreatic duct at the junction to the intestine. Excessive alcohol intake is the highest risk factor. Smoking cigarettes, overuse of medications like steroids, NSAIDS painkillers, blood pressure drugs like thiazides, and viral infections like mumps, hepatitis, and mononucleosis are also common factors in disease formation.

Prevention consists of avoiding the above risks. A low fat diet in four to five small meals a day together with good hydration is a basic requirement. Turmeric and ginger are effective in reducing the inflammation component and acupuncture can help with pain control, improved digestion and relaxation of the gastrointestinal musculature.

Liver disease, such as viral hepatitis, can result in nonfunctional liver cells, which allows for the accumulation of harmful toxins in the body that can lead to the failure of multiple organ systems. Liver damage can occur from the intake of excess sugar, especially fructose in the form of our modern high-fructose corn syrup (HFCS) which is found in many processed snacks and popular condiments, like ketchup. Excess alcohol intake, sodas, and some sports drinks can also affect liver function by adding too much sugar and fat to the blood. Monosodium glutamate (MSG) used in some packaged foods and many pasta and starchy dishes, hydrolysed vegetable oil, and yeast extracts can damage the liver. Herbs like comfrey for healing and pain relief, kava kava for anxiety, some antidepressants, and vitamin A in excess of 10,000 IU for too long a period of time have been associated with liver damage. The liver can be overwhelmed by too much of any ingestible item that may contain too high a concentration of substances deemed toxic to body cells.

Prevention consists of avoiding risky behavior involving illicit drugs, excess alcohol, smoking, vaccination against hepatitis A and B, attention to minimizing prescription drugs and only in recommended doses, avoiding inhalation of aerosol sprays, and maintaining a healthy weight, as obesity is strongly associated with liver disease. Liver toxins like alcohol, solvents, formaldehyde, pesticides, herbicides, and food additives can be removed or inhibited with milk thistle 500 mg daily, dandelion, parsley and a multivitamin with folate and vitamin B12. Foods like garlic, citrus (lemon, grapefruit) to flush out carcinogens and toxins, beets with flavonoids to improve function, leafy greens to neutralize metals, chemicals, and pesticides, green tea with catechins for liver function, avocado, and walnuts that enable the antioxidant, glutathione, for liver function, cruciferous vegetables that increase glucosinolates to create enzymes for digestion, turmeric that stimulates bile production to digest fats, and omega 3 for support of the liver for cleansing processes.

Diarrhea may be caused by viral, bacterial, fungal, and parasitic infections, emotional and physical stress, poor digestion, intolerance of certain food and medications, associated digestive disorders, chemotherapy, radiation, and non-specific bowel irritation.

Prevention is best accomplished by avoiding contact with infective microorganisms. Washing one's hands frequently and thoroughly especially when travelling and after preparing food, handling uncooked meat, using the toilet, sneezing, coughing, or blowing the nose is an effective deterrent. When washing is not readily available, using a hand sanitizer with at least 60 percent alcohol content is the next best thing. At home, try to thaw frozen items in a bowl of cold water in the fridge and not on the counter. Add lemon or lime to meats for initial seasoning and antimicrobial properties. When traveling in endemic areas, eat only hot cooked foods and fruit you peel yourself. Avoid washed, peeled fruit and cold vegetables, undercooked meats, suspicious dairy products, tap water, and drinks with ice cubes. Drink bottled water, beer, and wine in their original containers. Add probiotics to the diet at least twice daily to provide good bacteria and counteract the bad strains and especially while taking antibiotics. Avoid stressful situations, excess caffeine and alcohol, greasy, spicy, and fatty foods. Chew food thoroughly to enhance digestion and reduce the amount of undigested food reaching the colon. Evident diarrhea can be treated with natural products containing tannins with astringent (binding) properties, like guava, blackberry root bark, carob powder with applesauce and honey to soothe the intestine lining, bananas, rice and unbuttered toast. A soup with boiled potatoes, skinless chicken, cooked carrots, and plain brown rice, is well tolerated and healing.

Constipation refers to infrequent or difficulty emptying of the bowels usually due to hardened stool. Less than three bowel movements a week for any extended period of time, may lead to excessive straining, which may result in hemorrhoids. Risk factors include pregnancy, internal and external pressure, stress, and laxative abuse. An overindulgence in certain foods and fruit may also lead to constipation. An overuse of conventional synthetic stool softeners and bulk additives may lead to dependency, tolerance, and reduction of effect.

Prevention is simple. Drink lots of water and eat a diet high in fiber, vegetables, and whole grains. Stool consists largely of bacteria, and fiber promotes bacterial growth, which adds bulk and leads to a larger volume of stool, resulting in better bowel function. Basic high fiber stock includes beans, blueberries, cabbage, oats, peaches, prunes, and wheat germ. Aloe vera juice normalizes bowel function. Gentian root is a bitter herb that stimulates gastrointestinal activity. Angostura bitters with soda water before meals is recommended in cases without intestinal inflammation. Prune juice is a well-known popular remedy that starts peristalsis and should be taken with lots of water. Flaxseed, psyllium, senna, and triphala are natural laxatives that work by adding bulk to the stool. Probiotics, with a minimum of one billion organisms, serve to slow digestion, reduce excessive gas, and improve bowel efficiency. Avoidance of excess intake of dairy, red meat, and processed foods are essential to achieving relief.

Detoxification to rid the gastrointestinal system of industrial toxins, pesticides, drug deposits, food additives, heavy metals, environmental hormones, secondary smoke, and vapors that affect the normal genetics of cell growth, function, and immune response, damage organ systems and initiate and accelerate nerve degeneration. Protection and prevention against heavy metals can be promoted with a multivitamin with C and B complex and sulphur-containing products like garlic, onions, eggs, oat bran, pectin, and psyllium seeds. Calcium-D-glucarate, which is made in the body, can be added for chelation and removal of excess estrogens, LDL cholesterol, and plastic nanoparticles. A high-fiber diet can control unwanted bacteria, carcinogens, and excess yeast in the gut. Large doses of vitamin C can have an antibacterial and laxative effect. The major detoxification centers of the body are the skin, for heavy metal removal by sweating, the liver, for neutralization of bacterial, excess calcium, cholesterol, mercury, prescription drugs, and nicotine, with bile, the intestine, for removal of fat-soluble toxins, and the kidney, for removal of water-soluble toxins. The safest cleansing is with a weekly dose of lemon juice, extra virgin olive oil, and apple cider vinegar mix, one tablespoon, three times a day for one day. Others include fasting, three days a week, with only vegetable juices (cabbage and carrots) three times a day for three days. A high potency multivitamin with at least a 1,000mg of C should be added for support. A basic steam bath sauna pushes toxins out of the skin, with the addition of natural salts as a bonus toxin remover. All cleansing should include rebuilding of the contents of the intestines through proper nutrition.

Best Foods for Detoxification

Artichoke	Berries	Lemons	Watercress	Flaxseed
Apples	Brown rice	Ginger	Cabbage	Garlic

Hemorrhoids are swollen veins in the anal area, may be internal or external and are caused by too much pressure associated with straining during bowel movements. An increased incidence occurs during pregnancy, diarrhea or constipation and with obesity.

Prevention includes the addition of fiber, fruit, vegetables, and whole grains to your meals, drinking plenty of water to keep the urine a light yellow color, using stool softeners and creams of ointments containing witch hazel. Plenty of exercise can also help with more regular bowel movements.

Diseases of the Renal System

Kidney and bladder function are required for ridding the body of liquid waste material. Nephritis and cystitis are infections of the renal system that may not be evident until late in the disease, so that early detection and prevention take on even more importance. The onset of disease and its ultimate destruction resulting in renal failure is often associated with diabetes, hypertension, smoking, obesity, high cholesterol, age over sixty-five, inflammation, infections, and obstructions from stones, enlarged prostate, or cancers. Excess use of common painkillers like Ibuprofen, aspirin, naproxen, and other NSAIDS, can damage the kidneys. Conventional treatment in the early stages is with large doses of antibiotics for infections, laser or surgical removal of stones, and of renal failure with dialysis and/ or transplantation. *Avoid* excess intake of calcium and/ or oxalate-rich foods, like black tea, peanuts, spinach, strawberries, plus animal protein and sodas, as they are associated with a high incidence of stones.

Prevention is based on a diet of low oxalate foods, like Brussels sprouts and peas, low-fat milk, high-magnesium foods like avocado, broccoli, fish, and brown rice, high potassium foods like baked potato and dried apricot. Protein intake should be reduced to 10 percent and be only plant-based. Strict blood sugar control (A1C less than 7.0), blood pressure control (less than 130/80, and lipid control with LDL cholesterol less than 100, HDL more than 50, and triglycerides less than 150 md/dL. Blood pressure lowering medications like angiotensins and ACE inhibitors in these cases tend to be protective. Drinking plenty of water, between eight to ten glasses a day can prevent the concentration and accumulation of oxalates. Whether there is infection, stones, or outright disease, the intake of cranberries is the prevention and cure for most kidney problems. It contains high levels of antioxidants like flavonoids, flavonols, and anthocyanins, vitamins C and E, and magnesium, which are specific for promoting renal health. A handful of dried cranberries daily, one or two glasses of juice or capsules are effective in maintaining kidney function. Lemon juice, before meals and pure grade Epsom salts, one teaspoon at bedtime, alkalinizes the body to remove acid toxins that might be harmful. Turmeric with honey, *Plantago major* seeds (Llantén), cane piece senna (*Phyllanthus niruri*), dandelion (*Taxacum officinalis*), and baquiña contain antioxidants that help to prevent and dissolve early stones, by blocking the formation of oxalic acid compounds. One glass of apple juice with one teaspoon of apple cider vinegar introduces malic acid, which works like citric acid in lemon to raise the pH of the body to a more neutral, healthier level toward alkalinity.

Incontinence, the involuntary and unintentional loss of urine, can be associated with an overactive bladder, which could be nerve or stress-related, and result from low concentration of fluids (dehydration) as well as excess of fluids. Excess alcohol is dehydrating and also signals the brain to release urine. Caffeine-rich drinks and foods, citrus and pineapple with acids that can irritate the bladder, artificial sweeteners can trigger bladder symptoms, acidic condiments, prunes and dates with acids, processed foods with MSG and benzyll alcohol, and some blood pressure drugs that act as diuretics.

Prevention may be achieved by avoiding excesses, doing Kegel pelvic floor exercises to strengthen pelvic muscles, maintaining healthy weight levels, and stopping smoking, a source of toxic irritants, and preventing constipation, a major contributor.

Women's Health

Women's health issues are concerned with the natural promotion of hormonal and reproductive health, pregnancy and menopausal physiology, without resorting to powerful, sometimes toxic therapies. While general healthy and prenatal regimens should be followed closely, there are some strategic measures that are effective in preventing serious conditions and complications of natural events.

Dysmenorrhea, difficult or painful cramps during menstruation, is often associated with endometriosis, a condition where uterine tissue is found outside the uterus and subject to cyclic bleeding and abnormal scarring. As inflammation is the key component, natural prevention is directed at the reduction and regulation of the inflammatory response through an anti-inflammation diet of fresh whole fruit and vegetables, and reduction of high glycemic and processed foods. Black cohosh and goldenseal reduce inflammation and smooth muscle spasms, dong quai stimulates the uterus then relaxes it, and wild yam and motherwort both reduce muscle spasms. The effects of ginger in relieving gastrointestinal symptoms and chamomile in reducing anxiety and irritability are all well known.

Vaginitis is associated with the imbalance of bad vs. good bacteria, when there is an overgrowth of anaerobic bacteria (bad) and a reduction in lactobacilli (good). Yeast infection refers to the overgrowth of the fungus, *Candida albicans*, mainly due to excessive moisture. It is known as "thrush" when it occurs in the mouth, and can also be found in nail beds, skin folds, and as diaper rash. Trichomonas is a protozoan parasite that infects the vagina. Risk factors include risky sexual activity, hormonal changes, excess medications (antibiotics, steroids), overuse of hygienic products, excess douching, damp tight-fitting clothing and smoking.

Prevention and natural treatment include the addition of one to two cups of apple cider vinegar to bath water to increase the vaginal acidity that may kill anaerobic organisms and enable lactobacilli to thrive. Yogurt may be added directly to the vaginal area three times a day until the symptoms are gone. Tea tree oil in warm water may be applied three times daily to kill fungi and bacteria. A combination of fenugreek powder and milk applied to the vagina may raise the pH level, boost the immune system and add good lactobacilli.

Pregnancy and menopause are not diseases but normal physiological processes and will be included here for purposes of providing information on successful outcomes. Pregnancy is the condition most in need of the perfect health profile. Weight, vital signs, electrolytes, blood components, and all organ systems must be in top condition to ensure a natural progression, successful delivery, and healthy outcome.

Foods That Benefit Pregnancy

Eggs (protein & choline)	Salmon (omega 3)	Beans (protein & fiber)	Sweet potatoes
Whole grains (fiber & selenium)	Walnuts (fiber, protein & plant-based omega3)	Yogurt (calcium & probiotics)	Leafy greens (vitamins, folate, & minerals)
Lean meats	Fruit (*berries)	Citrus (vitamin C & D)	Water

Foods to Avoid during Pregnancy

Raw meat (infection)	Raw seafood	Deli meats (listeria)	Oceanfish with mercury
Smoked seafood	Lakefish with PCBs	Raw shellfish (vibrio)	Raw eggs
Soft cheeses	Paté (listeria to baby)	Caffeine (diuresis)	Alcohol (development)

The list is long: no mackerel, swordfish, canned chunk light tuna, sushi, lox, kippers, bluefish, striped bass, pike, trout, walleye salmon, oysters, clams, mussels, Caesar dressings, mayonnaise, homemade ice cream, custards, hollandaise sauces, brie, camembert, Roquefort, feta, gorgonzola (may be unpasteurized milk), or unwashed vegetables, will greatly reduce the chances of contracting unwanted viral or bacterial infections..

Postpartum hemorrhage is the most serious and feared complication resulting from the failure of the uterus to contract normally after the delivery process. This may be associated with prolonged labor, infection, or obstructions. Conventional treatment involves oxytocin (Pitocin). Natural prevention involves prenatal lowering of the cholesterol levels, a reduction in obesity, and the addition of calcium and magnesium to enable and promote uterine contractibility. Angelica root is a well-known uterine stimulant used to extract the remnants of the placenta. Calcium-rich botanicals include red raspberry leaf, sesame seeds, spinach, collard greens, blackstrap molasses, and the dairy milk and yogurt. After delivery, breastfeeding itself stimulates hormone release for uterine contraction as well as massaging until a firm ball is felt. The botanicals, blue cohosh, witch hazel and Shepherd's purse, a potent coagulant and vasoconstrictor, have been used as tinctures taken sublingually, to stop the bleeding. They should not be used during pregnancy. Elevation of the feet and application of ice packs should also be used. Depression and anxiety during and after pregnancy have been associated with a deficiency of omega 3 fatty acids, particularly EPA and DHA, and serotonin, a principal neurotransmitter. Replacement fish oils and SAMe (S-adenosyl methionine) can be taken, along with folic acid as a stabilizer. Fatigue, hair and nail thinning, and dry skin, possible symptoms of hypothyroidism or thyroiditis, may be prevented with adequate selenium from nuts and vegetables, turmeric to reduce concomitant inflammation and realign autoimmunity and probiotics to regulate the digestive processes. Healing and coping mechanisms should be examined and promoted on the emotional level.

Menopause is the condition that occurs naturally over the age of fifty, when there is a decline in the levels of estrogen and DHEA-S in the blood and body tissues. Estrone and progesterone from the uterus normally remain. The symptoms of hot flashes, night sweats, mood swings, vaginal dryness, sleep disturbances, nausea, dry eyes, memory lapses, palpitations, incontinence, headaches, depression, anxiety, decreased libido, joint pains, and weight gain, are well known. Conventional treatment is with various combinations of hormone replacement therapy (HRT), which substantially reduce the symptoms but increase the risk of estrogenic cancers, deep vein thrombosis and stroke, and gall bladder disease. Though the risk is listed at 5/1,000, it is still significant.

Prevention and treatment of excessive symptoms with natural therapies begin with the establishment and pursuit of a regular regimen of physical activity. A solid aerobic workout (walking, running, swimming, gym) directed at strength, flexibility, and balance training is strongly recommended. In addition to the weight loss factor and vital signs, the endorphin release system is essential to the proper regulation of menopause.

Adequate sleep is important for physiologic function. Warm milk, chamomile and lemon balm tea, valerian 160 to 300 mg or melatonin 3 to 10 mg at bedtime are effective and safe. Nutritional support in the form of total elimination of processed and refined foods (white sugar, rice, flour), sodas, artificial sweeteners, and animal fats, and the incorporation of adequate water intake of eight to ten glasses daily, foods high in omega 3 fatty acids, two to four daily servings of soy with isoflavones which are protective against estrogenic problems, calcium 1,000 to 1,500 mg as citrate in between or carbonate with meals, magnesium 300 to 600 mg, vitamin D 400 to 800 IU or fifteen minutes sunshine daily, and a multivitamin with B complex and vitamin C 200-500 mg.

Hot flashes can be controlled with black cohosh 20 to 80 mg twice daily, red clover 500 mg, evening primrose oil 500 to 1000 mg up to three times a day, vitamin E 400 to 800 IU, and sage and alfalfa. Vitex (Chastetree berries) are effective in cases of lingering menstrual irregularities and ginkgo biloba teas increases cerebral blood flow to help the memory.

Vaginal dryness is due to thinning, shortening and loss of elasticity of the lining, reduced collagen, atrophy of glands, less blood supply, higher acidity, and decreased presence of good lactobacilli, all contributing to a decrease in sexual activity which further exacerbates the symptoms. Prevention and natural treatment consists of increasing the pH in the lining to a more acceptable alkaline level, damiana (*Turnera diffusa*) and papaya (*Carica p.*) with natural phytoestrogens can restore some moisture, and panax ginseng 100 to 200 mg daily for two to three months at a time, can restore some libido by increasing the normal adrenal cortisol and DHEA levels.

Depression and anxiety are can be approached with St. John's wort 300 mg three times daily or Schizandra chinensis, a fruit that is effective in controlling the irritability and insomnia of menopause. Mind-body relaxing breathing techniques, massage, energy medicine, journaling, guided imagery, meditation, yoga, tai chi, qi qong, and aromatherapy, all have evidence-based support for reducing menopausal symptoms.

Close regulation of blood pressure, blood sugar, and cholesterol levels are essential to reducing the risk of common conditions like polycystic ovary, eclampsia, and fibroids.

Men's Health

Men's health issues focus on conditions encountered primarily during middle and old age. **Erectile dysfunction**, a component of impotence, affects approximately 40 percent of men over the age of forty, 50 percent over fifty, and so on. The causes have been attributed to low testosterone levels as a result of increasing age, diabetes, low cholesterol, and testes dysfunction, as well as blockage of blood flow to the penile tissue, and malfunction of the nerve stimulation mechanism required to initiate and maintain the blood flow stages involved. Conventional treatment is aimed at testosterone replacement with human chorionic gonadotropin (HCG), DHEA, which may lead to muscle cramping, tumors and liver damage, and sildenafil- (Viagra) like compounds that work by inhibition of enzymes that affect nitric oxide and its effect on smooth muscle tissue that directs blood flow, which may lead to increased red blood cells, blood clots, heart attacks, stroke and prostatic hypertrophy. The newer selective androgen receptor modulators (S a.m. are effective and have fewer side effects.

Prevention and maintenance through the use of natural testosterone enhancers have been utilized around the world for centuries. Pure pomegranate juice and fenugreek powder increase testosterone levels without side effects. Panax ginseng improves testosterone levels, reduces oxidative stress and promotes smooth muscle function. Zinc in oysters, shellfish, raw milk, cheese, and yogurt aids in testosterone production. Vitamin D, known as the steroid hormone, increases testosterone, maintains semen quality and boosts sperm count. The amino acid, arginine, in pistachio nuts enhances the relaxation of smooth muscles. The nitrates in dark leafy green vegetables, and the antioxidants in ginkgo biloba, watermelon rind, cranberries, peanuts, grapefruit, onions, chocolate, beets, tuna, salmon and herbal teas, all act as vasodilators to help to increase blood circulation. Exercise directed at reduction of body fat through high intensity short sessions together with intermittent fasting to boost insulin, leptin, adiponectin and cholecystokinin levels, helps to potentiate testosterone activity. *Caution* must be taken to keep testosterone levels commensurate with and appropriate to age, as abnormally high levels are associated with androgenic cancers. A reduction in the reaction to stress serves to keep cortisol release under control so as to allow the testosterone present to have effect. Chronic stress is strongly associated with loss of libido.

Benign prostatic hypertrophy is the enlargement of the prostate gland associated with the production of 5-alpha reductase enzyme that produce excess abnormal testosterone (DHT), inflammation and semen retention. The risk factors include age over fifty, family history, diabetes, heart diseases, a use of beta blocker medications, obesity, and lack of physical activity.

Prevention is centered on the promotion of prostate health through dietary strategies. Cooked tomatoes release the antioxidants, lycopene, and selenium, which factors in the promotion of prostate health. Fruit like pomegranate with ellagitannins, plants with beta sitosterol and pumpkin seed oil reduce the formation of DHT. Cruciferous vegetables, like broccoli, cabbage, cauliflower and kale, contain indole-3-carbinols which reduce inflamed prostate tissue. Whole soy foods contain genistein, which improves prostate metabolism. Fish with monounsaturated omega 3 fatty acids and fiber to avoid constipation are both protective. Saw palmetto (*Serenoa repens*) promotes healthy function and can reduce a swollen, inflamed prostate. *Pygeum africanum*, stinging nettle (*Urtica dioica*), turmeric, and ginger all have positive effects on the inflammation response. Daily exercise in the form of vigorous walking, jogging, biking, or hiking three to four times a week promotes a healthy circulation, boosts immunity, reduces inflammation and increases healing. *Avoid* the intake of processed foods, saturated and trans-fats, red meat, alcohol and caffeine as excesses may lead to increases in urgency, frequency of urination and bladder inflammation. A healthy prostate lowers the risk of developing cancer in the later years.

Skin

The promotion of healthy skin using natural products is widely accepted and available. Almost all have been tested and offer various degrees of relief and healing properties. The ingestion of fruit with high fiber content and skin healing properties, like pomegranate, chamomile and green tea, and certain mushrooms are complement to the use of soaps, lotions, and creams.

Argan oil from a Moroccan fruit tree is rich in vitamin E and effective against eczema, psoriasis, wrinkles, and dry skin. Aloe vera gel contains over one hundred phytochemicals among which is the best moisturizer, acetomannan. Soy prevents abnormal pigmentation in that it can fade brown spots of aging and sun damage. Licorice, mulberry, burberry, citrus fruit with high levels of vitamin C are all effective skin healers. Maitake mushrooms (*Grifola frondosa*) have strong antioxidant properties that promote collagen repair of human skin fibroblasts that can improve rosacea and redness. Topical chamomile, oatmeal, licorice, and cucumber extracts, all soothe dry tender skin and promote healing. Rhodiola crenulata treatments can reduce the incidence of metastasis of skin melanomas and applications offer a degree of protection to sensitive skin. Coffee-berry, the outer rind of the coffee bean, is high in antioxidant activity for prevention and reduction of wrinkles, fine skin lines, and brown age spots. Grapes, red wine with resveratrol, a polyphenol antioxidant and anti-inflammatory agent, green tea extract with catechins, all protect the skin against excess ultraviolet radiation.

Acne consists of pimples, cysts, nodules of sebaceous glands at the base of hair follicles, which become filled with oil and dead skin cells, which lead to plugged pores, especially on the face, neck, chest, back, and shoulders. These sores may or may not become infected and/or inflamed and are exacerbated by overstimulation by androgenic hormones from the adrenal glands of both males and females occurring mainly during puberty and teenage years. Risk factors include positive family history, contact with oily or greasy substances like lotions and creams, grease in the work area, friction by items like cell phones, helmets, and tight collars, emotional stress and physical squeezing may worsen the lesions but is not considered as a direct cause. The toxins from smoking being eliminated by the skin can cause clogging. It is a global skin disease with a long history of multiple treatments, one of which was to apply a thin layer of hot bees wax to the face. It often worked but was very uncomfortable and cumbersome to maintain. Current conventional treatment leans toward facial ablation with lasers, chemical abrasives, antibiotics and corticosteroids. Further treatment is required to alleviate the resultant scarring.

Prevention begins with a dietary adjustment to *avoid* high fat dairy and carbohydrates (especially junk food), chocolate, drugs containing corticosteroids and androgens (like muscle-building enhancers), or lithium. Instead, increase consumption of fresh fruits and vegetables, preferably organic and local, lots of fiber to take in zinc, vitamins A, C, and E that reduce inflammation. Basic skin hygiene should be sensible, with the use of gentle products that keep the pores open and functional, rather than clogged with the residue of heavy oils and creams. For oily skin, use an astringent that contains alcohol, witch hazel or salicylic acid, to reduce oil production and tighten pores. For sensitive skin, use a water-based cleanser with chamomile or rosewater, and vitamin B derivatives like pantheol, to lock in the moisture. Where possible, use oil-free, hypoallergenic make-up bases, and remove regularly.

Tea tree oil, one drop applied to affected area three times a day, disinfects pores and kills bacteria, fungi, and viruses. Baking soda is a good antiseptic that unplugs pores, removes dead skin cells, regulates pH balance upward toward alkalinity, and reduces inflammation. A mixture with warm water into a paste is applied, left in place for twenty minutes, and then rinsed. Oregon grape root and oatmeal clean the pores, absorb excess oil, remove dead skin cells and exhibit antimicrobial activity. Lemon contains citric acid which cleans dirt from pores, hardens the oils, and removes dead skin cells. Use two to three times a week and leave it on for one to two hours, then rinse, as daily usage may lead to over drying of the skin. As with all external lemon products, caution must be taken as exposure to excessive sunlight may lead to hyperpigmentation (photo-dermatitis). Aloe vera gel is one of the best moisturizers known. In addition to being antibacterial, antiviral and antifungal, it blocks bacteria from infecting acne lesions, and promotes good healing.

Herpes simplex virus infection in an infant or a child is usually by direct contact with an adult, may be oral or genital from the birth canal. Later viral transmission may be by common utensils usage, kissing, sharing lip balm, and sexual activity. The first infection is usually mild, with the first recurrence being more obvious and symptomatic. Risk factors include associated stress trigger mechanisms, both emotional and physical, a weakened or compromised immune system, female gender, and multiple sexual partners. Sores occurring mostly on the mouth are type 1, and sores on the genitals are type 2. Infection is for life.

Conventional treatment is with antiviral medications, like acyclovir, famciclovir, and valacyclovir, oral and/or topical daily until controlled.

Prevention is obviously directed at the avoidance of initial contact with an infected person is of primary importance. Recurrences can be reduced by strengthening the immune system to modulate the response to stressors, through dietary measures and use of enhancers like shiitake mushrooms when possible and astragalus bark daily. Echinacea can be taken for acute attacks up to three times daily for three days. Cat's claw tonic and kelp (seaweed) are recommended for regular use. A diet high in lysine-rich amino acids , like fish, chicken, beef, lamb, milk, cheese, beans, fruit and vegetables, and yogurt; and low in argine-rich foods like chocolate, coconut, oats, wheat and soy, is recommended. Propolis, a resin made by bees, has antioxidants that help fight herpes infection and boosts immunity, may be applied topically or taken orally. And the application of lemon balm cream three times a day, along with honey, aloe vera gel, and calendula oil may help soften and heal crusted sores. Astragalus potentiates the action of acyclovir.

Eczema, a type of atopic dermatitis, is manifested as dry itchy inflamed patches on the scalp, elbows, hands, knees and ankles, associated with chronic allergies and long-term recurrent inflammation. Specific substances in the diet and environment are usually involved. This dermatitis is increasingly seen as a skin barrier disease, which facilitates the entry of allergens that cause successive allergies in the gut, nasal mucosa, mouth, and eyes. Conventional treatment with steroid pills, creams and ointments may cause an unwanted thinning of the skin. Immune system modulators like pimecrolimus and tacrolimus may become tolerant and lead to side effects as well.

Natural treatments with continuous moisturizers like warm, tepid baths, and showers using bland soaps, hypoallergenic after-bath moisturizers, over the counter anti-itch lotions to reduce mechanical scratching, and low potency steroid creams may give effective results. A strict anti-inflammation diet with avoidance of all pro-inflammation products is recommended. The GAP (gut and psychology syndrome) diet that focuses on foods, like bone broth, fermented cod liver oil, and probiotics, that soothe and heal the gut lining so that good bacteria and immune system healing nutrients can be absorbed has given good results. Supplementing with GLA (gamma linolenic acid), an omega 3 fatty acid found in evening primrose oil, black currant and borage oil, at 500 mg taken twice daily can nourish the skin, hair, and nails. *Avoiding* possible allergens like gluten (wheat), casein (milk), refined sugars, and white rice, as well as psychological stressors can reduce the incidence of attacks. The topical application of aloe vera gel, calendula, or chaparral oil or lotion, coconut oil to the scalp, sea spray with salt and magnesium, and Epsom salt baths, can give some relief.

Psoriasis is a painful, sometimes fatal disorder that is associated with the breakdown or malfunction of the immune system, where T cells attack healthy skin cells by mistake. The reaction changes the normal life cycle of skin cells resulting in an accumulation of extra skin cells forming thick silvery scales and dry itchy red patches. Trigger mechanisms include cold weather, emotional stress, infections, smoking, heavy alcohol consumption; medications like beta blockers for high blood pressure, anti-malarials, and the iodides. Risk factors are a positive family history, frequent viral and bacterial infections that further weaken the immune system, high stress levels, obesity as the plaques may develop in the skin folds and creases. Smoking initiates and increases the severity of the disease. It is associated also with diabetes, eye inflammations, joint arthritis, cardiovascular disease, metabolic syndrome of hypertension, high cholesterol, and high insulin levels, and other autoimmune diseases like celiac disease, multiple sclerosis, inflammatory bowel disease, kidney disease, and Parkinson's.

Conventional treatment is with corticosteroids and other strong immune system suppressants. Treatment with a narrow band of ultraviolet radiation may be used along with adjunctive medications to control the scale production.

Prevention and natural treatment is supportive, by keeping the skin moist with aloe vera gel, petroleum jelly, olive oil, and coconut oil. Pat the skin dry after a bath, then apply the remedy. Avoid rubbing with a rough towel. Bathe with care, using lukewarm water to which salts or fine oatmeal has been added. Soak. Reduction in the frequency of baths could help to maintain the natural body oils. Exposure to small doses of ultraviolet radiation of the sun is a good treatment for psoriasis (twenty minutes a day, three days a week). Overexposure may make it worse. Tar products as creams and gels, enhance the positive effects of sun exposure. Cessation of smoking and alcohol consumption is beneficial to the immune system and general health.

Vitiligo is the loss of pigment in the skin (leukoderma) due to the destruction or malfunction of the pigment-forming cells (melanocytes). It affects all skin colors with equal frequency. Effects are largely cosmetic. The most common successful conventional treatment is with a combination of ultraviolet phototherapy to induce pigment cells to produce melanin, plus synthetic drugs, afamelanotides, with positive results in only a few months. There is no known successful prevention to date. Natural treatments for which scientific evidence exists include a mixture of neem oil, milk ghee, turmeric, and honey, which in ayurvedic medicine, kills off the remaining pigmented cells, leaving the entire skin bleached white. Restoration of pigment can be done through surgical skin grafts, pigment promoting chemicals and natural products like ginkgo biloba which performed better than placebo. Ficus carica (figs) leaves contain both psoralens and bergaptene, which are effective in restoring skin pigmentation in vitiligo, psoriasis and alopecia. A preparation can be used topically or orally. PUVA is a combination of psoralens and ultraviolet A long wavelength radiation, which is effective in slowing the progression severe skin diseases.

Alopecia, or baldness outside of genetic patterns, is caused by loss of hair follicles associated with aging, clogged oil glands, hormonal changes, iron and protein deficiencies, rapid weight loss, excessive vitamin A consumption, scalp infection, birth control pills (estrogens), menopause, thyroid disorders, excessive use of drying or tightening hair machines, use of chemicals, and anabolic steroids. Abnormal non-genetic patchy hair loss is known as alopecia areata in both men and women. Male baldness is a genetic anatomic pattern of scaly follicles predisposed to destruction by androgenic hormones.

Prevention and treatment are more effective when the process is in the early stages. remedies for which there is ample evidence include the use of aloe vera gel (not juice), massaged gently in daily, so that its enzymes, oils and anti-inflammatory phytochemicals and moisturizers could improve scalp health, open clogged follicles, and slow hair loss. Evening primrose (*Oenthera bienis*) and sesame oil, both essential fatty acids, stimulate hair follicles and improve dry scaly skin in alopecia. Leave a mixture on overnight and rinse out in the morning. Rosemary (*Rosmarinus officinalis*) is rich in volatile oils, camphor, borneol, camphene, cineol, and pineol, which when mixed into a lotion, applied at bedtime, covered with a shower cap, rinsed in the morning, stimulates hait bulbs and follicles to renewed activity that reduces premature baldness. A mixture of onion, cinnamon, beeroot leaves, and turmeric in warm water can control chronic recurrent scalp infections. A decoction of hibiscus flowers, geranium and amaranth leaves is good for preventing baldness through promotion of hair health. The addition of copious amounts of spinach, lettuce and gooseberry juice to the diet supplies a generous amount of antioxidants for hair repair and rejuvenation.

Mouth

Pharyngitis, or sore throat, refers to an inflammation of the pharynx, usually associated with viral infections which tend to be self-limited or bacterial infections like Streptococcus, which may require antibiotics. If the symptoms of scratchiness and difficulty swallowing are accompanied by fever lasting more than a week, it is more likely of bacterial origin. Risk factors include dryness, allergies, irritants (tobacco smoke, household chemicals), muscle strain (yelling or talking too much), GERD when acids back up into the throat and cause burns, frequent sinusitis, decreased immunity, HIV infections, and tumors.

Prevention and natural treatment highlights the warm saltwater gargle that breaks up and expels secretions. Licorice root and slippery elm gargles are also effective. Marshmallow root tea introduces a soothing mucus-like gel to the mucosal surface and honey and lemon tea provides antibiotic and antiviral activity as well as calming a raw cough. A combination of echinacea and sage spray is just as soothing as chlorhexidrine /lidocaine. Peppermint has menthol and eugenol which help to thin mucus, calm a cough, open stuffy passages, reduce inflammation, and convey antibacterial and antiviral activities.

Gingivitis, or gum disease, is an early form of periodontitis, which occurs when the gums pull away from the teeth and the infection spreads to include the bone and connective tissues. Poor mouth hygiene can be associated with diabetes and a weak immune system that allows pathogenic bacteria in plaque, tartar. and calculus to remain on the teeth, then penetrate the gums, the immune system response plays a definitive role in how far the disease will progress. Oral infection contributes to atherosclerosis and coronary heart disease particularly in men over the age of sixty-five.

Prevention measures include flossing daily after every meal and before brushing at night. Brush your teeth a minimum of two times daily with baking soda and unrefined sea salt to cleanse the area and neutralize the acids in the mouth and make it more alkaline. Rinse with an antibacterial gargle that is gentle and can be used often. Note that washes with chlorhexadrine may stain the tooth enamel so should not be used for more than a week at a time. Chewing a raw garlic clove conveys all the antibiotic, antiviral, and antifungal power of allicin to disinfect and clean the oral cavity. Avoid refined processed sugars, sodas, white rice, and white bread. Pathogenic bacteria thrive on these media. Stop smoking as the toxins build up too much carbon and free radicals and contribute to chemical reactions that remove required minerals and vitamins. Reduce stress to increase immunity to fight the huge numbers of bacteia in the mouth. The following botanicals are known to improve oral health by natural means. Oak bark is high in tannins, antioxidants, and minerals that act as astringents to tighten tissues, strengthen blood vessels, reduce inflammation, and along with yarrow, stimulate blood clotting agents to prevent frequent bleeding. Coconut oil, St. John's wort and silver fir extract have antibacterial activity. Pine tree extract, chamomile tea, nettles, and greater celandine prevent disease through their antioxidant, antiseptic, and immune boosting properties. Any mouthwash containing the volatile oils of the mints, menthol, thymol, eugenol, and eucalyptol, are effective in oral hygiene.

Dental caries are holes in the teeth that occur when the structure breaks down, decays, and is eroded by pathogenic bacteria that produce acids that destroy the enamel. These bacteria thrive in an acid medium and on nutrients provided mostly by sugars.

Prevention, according to Center for Disease Control recommendations, includes routine and regular hygiene by brushing twice daily with a fluoride toothpaste and flossing after each meal to remove food particles. Eat a balanced diet and make regular dental visits. Natural products containing the phytochemicals, catechol, emetine, quinine and flavones, found green tea, aloe vera, cinchona bark, soy and many beans and vegetables of the plant families, Polygonum, Rhamnus and Senna, have activity against oral cavity bacteria like *Streptococcus mutans*. Extracts with tannins, alkaloids, and flavonoids from the leaves of witch hazel, cloves of garlic, and propolis resin from bees, exhibit similar properties.

Nose

Sinusitis is the inflammation, congestion of the mucosal lining and accumulation of mucus in the sinus cavities. It may involve the nasal, maxillary, ethmoidal, or frontal sinuses and be due to viral, bacterial, fungal , parasitic, or allergic responses to external pollutants like cigarette smoke and industrial chemicals, intranasal drug use, trauma, anatomic deviations, polyps, associated asthma, weakened immunity, and/or overuse of decongestants or other medications like aspirin sensitivity. Rhinitis, stuffy nose, is the inflammation of the nasal mucosa due mainly to allergies and common cold. Conventional treatments are administrated with decongestants, antihistamines, corticosteroids and antibiotics. *Avoid* using sprays and inhalers more than three times a day for three days continuously.

Natural proven remedies include humidification of the air, use of cleansing filters regularly to reduce mold, breathing vaporizers (steam) to reduce swollen nasal passages, warm heat (wet towel application), basal saline solution flush with salt water, general hydration that thins mucus, and decreasing alcohol intake. Effective botanicals include peppermint and eucalyptus inhalation. Bromelain in pineapples reduces nasal swelling. Apple cider vinegar, three tablespoons per cup of hot water, three times daily will thin out and expel mucus. Vitamin C, omega 3 fish, and oregano oils boost immunity. Cayenne pepper spray reduces nasal obstruction and sensitivity. Soup with garlic, onions, cayenne, and horseradish dissolve and thin mucus and provide antibiotic actions. Grapefruit seed extract nasal spray has antibacterial, antiviral, antifungal, and anti-parasitic activity.

Ears

The most common ear infection is **otitis media**, infection of the middle ear, the air-filled space located behind the eardrum. Due to bacteria or viruses that also affect the Eustachian tubes, nose, and throat, it mostly affect infants and children exposed to group infections, seasonal factors, and poor air quality. It is manifested by pain, fever, loss of balance, drainage of fluid from the ear, possible hearing loss.

Conventional treatments is with antibiotics, though many ear infections have no bacterial basis. Some 80 percent of these infections improve on their own, the overuse of antibiotics cause resistant strains and more serious infections by removing the good bacteria as well. Antibiotics should be used if there is a fever over 102°F along with other signs.

Prevention is directed at maintaining good hygiene of the ear passage by removal of earwax when present in abundance. Introduction of Q tips into the ear canal is discouraged to avoid injury to the eardrum and lining and as it may push earwax deeper. Use of a suction device is better. Inserting a cotton ball wet with white vinegar and alcohol into the outer part of the canal, tilting the head up then back down to allow drainage is another good way to remove impacted wax. Dietary measures to prevent ear infections include breastfeeding (colostrum) to build immunity against colds and respiratory allergies. Probiotics will build good bacteria and result in less intestinal and throat infections. Colloidal silver is a natural antibiotic, black elderberry syrup provides antioxidant cell protection from airborne elements. Olive leaf extract provides basic immune support against viral, fungal and bacterial pathogens, and echinacea can be used for acute attacks of runny nose, cough, and earache. Herbal steam inhalation with thyme oil twice daily will help the clear the passages, nasal, Eustachian and ear congestion.

Hearing loss occurs when the nerve of the inner ear and /or the bones of the middle ear are injured or otherwise incapacitated from repeated trauma, noise, infections, clogged ear canals from impacted wax, or genetic predisposition. Water in the ear from swimming or showering when in contact with earwax makes it swell.

Prevention is best achieved through avoidance and use of protection devices like earplugs and earmuffs. Noise levels greater than the eighty-eight decibel threshold, like hairdryers, lawnmowers, headphones, MP3, iPods, cell phones, garbage disposals, and grinders need to be avoided.

Adding omega 3 fatty acids from cold water fish to the diet strengthens blood vessels in the ear sensory system. Vitamin D and folic acid from adequate sunshine exposure, fortified dairy, spinach, asparagus, broccoli, beans, eggs and nuts, provide antioxidant protection for nerve tissue of the inner ear and repair of DNA cellular damage. Magnesium from bananas, potatoes, artichokes and broccoli, zinc from dark chocolate, oysters, and turkey, vitamin C and glutathione from citrus fruit and bell peppers, protect from noise induced nerve tissue damage.

Tinnitus is the perceived sound when there is no external source and consists of ringing or buzzing in the ears. It is a very common affecting greater than fifty million people in the USA. It is associated with head or neck injury, overuse of high dose NSAIDS like ibuprofen 800 mg, three times a day for weeks to months, and cardiovascular disease involving the vascular blood flow to the ears.

Conventional treatment may be with a combination of cochlear implants and psychological counseling and the addition of neutralizing sounds.

Prevention involves reducing volume and frequency of exposure to loud noises and reducing the use of chewy foods that may act as triggers. To maintain ear health through dietary measures, vitamin B12, and zinc support nerve tissue, ginkgo biloba is good for blood flow in small vessels, the antioxidant activity of pomegranate is protective against toxic nerve damage, and the intake of almonds to increase red blood cells and decrease cholesterol to improve blood flow.

Eyes

Prevention of glaucoma, diabetic retinopathy, and delay of cataract and age-related macular degeneration would be a major advancement in health care by greatly reducing the incidence and prevalence of blindness, prolonging productivity, and improving the quality of life of the global population.

Regular physical exercise increases the blood flow to small vessels and improves eye health tremendously. The provision of adequate nutrients to the nerve cells of the retina and optic nerve is supported by promoting heart health through the reduction of cholesterol levels, prevention of atherosclerosis, and normalization of blood pressure. A diet rich in antioxidants supports the cellular integrity of all the eye tissues. Citrus fruit with vitamin C and antioxidants, fresh vegetables like spinach provide carotenoids for cataract prevention; bilberry, blueberry with zinc, lutein, zeaxanthin, astaxanthin for age-related macular degeneration; apricots, broccoli, cantaloupe, carrots to provide beta-carotene for vitamin A for the health of retinal cells; grapes, sweet potatoes, and red wine to provide pycnogenol and resveratrol; and walnuts with omega 3 fatty acids and melatonin. All protect the eye tissues against malfunction and premature degeneration. When fresh whole food is not available or when extra nutrients are deemed necessary, supplements with the full complement of eye vitamins, like Areds formula II, are recommended.

Cataract formation occurs with injury to the natural lens or changes in the metabolic pathways that lead to disruption of the protein, resulting in clouding and decreased vision. Risk factors include onset at age over forty with maturity around age sixty, congenital genetic mutation, chemicals, diabetes, excess alcohol consumption associated with malnutrition, obesity, and arthritis associated with chronic inflammation, ultraviolet B radiation exposure, corticosteroid use and adverse effects of other medications. Cataracts have been associated with deficiencies of vitamin C, carotenoids (vitamin A based), disruptions in the sorbitol pathway involved in diabetes, the organic compounds, N-acetyl histidine, N-acetyl carnitine, and acetyl-1-carnitine, magnesium, and celiac disease with malabsorption of micronutrients like lanosterol, fisetin and the omega 3 fatty acid, alpha lipoic acid.

Conventional treatment is being skeptical on all prevention methods, and doing surgery with implants in the early stages.

Prevention is logical by at least attempting to correct these deficiencies. Start by reducing excess exposure to UV radiation by using protective sunglasses as needed. Avoid eye injury and overuse of steroids and synthetic medications. Maintain a healthy balanced diet that contains ample antioxidants from fresh fruit and vegetables with carotenoids, like spinach and broccoli, green tea, grapes, bilberry and all berries, onions, garlic, and Brazil nuts with selenium. Eye vitamins with A, C, and E, lutein, zeaxanthin and zinc are recommended. In cases of early cataract formation, some positive results have been seen with the application of botanicals antioxidant and inhibitory activity, like chrysanthemum, cineraria maritima, grapeseed extract, cloves with eugenol, black pepper with piperidine, ginger with gingerols, garlic with allicin and organosulfuraphanes.

Glaucoma is a neurodegenerative disease of the optic nerve and retinal ganglion cells that is associated with impaired flow of intraocular fluid, reduced ocular blood microcirculation, oxidative stress at the mitochondrial level resulting in high intraocular pressure. Risk factors include age over forty, family history, ethnicity (African Americans and Hispanics), diabetes, obesity associated with inflammation and poor health, heart disease, hypertension with impaired blood perfusion, hypothyroidism, injury, long-term intake of corticosteroids, and other unhealthy eye conditions.

Conventional treatment is directed at intraocular pressure control and neuroprotection with oral medications, topical drops, laser, surgery stents and anatomic manipulations to achieve a level below 20 mmHg. Early detection and pressure control reduces but does not stop the progression to vision loss.

Prevention should be directed at maximizing the efficiency of the microcirculation by improving blood vessel linings, keeping the cardiovascular system functional, maintaining the optic nerve integrity and reducing the eye pressure to within an individual target range. Dietary antioxidants will reduce the presence of damaging free radical and reactive oxygen species of oxidative stress at the mitochondrial level. Through whole foods, citrus juices, fresh carrots, spinach, collards, and kale, which contain ample amounts of vitamin A, both alpha and beta carotene, visual pigments like cryptoxanthin, zeaxanthin, lutein and astaxanthin, and minerals like zinc, potassium, magnesium, selenium, and chromium. Supplementing with Coenzyme Q 10, 90 to 200 mg capsule daily will help with DNA repair and omega 3 fish oils 1,000 mg daily offer nerve and connective tissue protection. Botanicals for glaucoma include ginkgo biloba at a dosage of 60 mg of 24 percent, daily in capsules or tea, for good blood flow in small vessels. Saffron extract at 100 mg a day, is an expensive antioxidant that lowers intraocular pressure. *Cannabis sativa* and derivatives have been shown to lower eye pressure but the delivery system needs to be optimized to reduce the side effects and frequency of use. Exercising three times a week, thirty minutes a day, increases the release endorphins, lowers intraocular pressure, improves blood flow, and protects the optic nerve through improved perfusion.

Macular degeneration is the deterioration and loss of the cone cells of the retina that are responsible for central and color vision needed for reading, driving and distinguishing fine details. The wet form involves the presence of blood beneath the macula and is more progressive. Age is the most important risk factor, as the condition has a higher incidence in the over sixty-five age group. Though the exact cause of cell death is as yet unknown, there is a strong association with nutritional deficiencies as in an unhealthy diet deficient in antioxidants, especially the carotenoid visual pigments, lutein, zeaxanthin and astaxanthin, smoking (toxins), positive family history, ethnic Caucasians, obesity with inflammation, cardiovascular diseases with hypertension and high cholesterol levels. As the result of oxidative stress, toxins accumulate in the macular cells, thereby drawing in more inflammatory response leading to cell death and entry of abnormal blood vessels, which bleed and lead to scarring and total dysfunction.

Conventional treatments include nutritional improvement with antioxidants, plus laser and eye injections of chemicals that help absorb hemorrhage and reduce the formation of new fragile blood vessels.

Prevention is directed at maintaining a healthy balanced diet of fresh fruit and vegetables, additional antioxidant intake of lutein 10 to 20 mg and zeaxanthin 2 mg in berries, B vitamins in spinach, kale and collards, minerals like zinc 10 mg, copper 2 mg, chromium and magnesium, flavonoids in red wine, chocolate, and omega 3 fish oils and nuts, and cessation of smoking.

The retinopathy encountered in diabetes destroys the eye tissues by repeated hemorrhages and plasma leakage and subsequent destructive scarring. Strict blood sugar control is required to prevent blindness. The use of cinnamon, gymnema silvestre, and garlic can help with maintaining control.

References for Chapter 4 (NHDP)

1. Diet and risk of leukemia in the women's health study. Ross JA, et al. (2002) Cancer Epidemiol. Biomarkers Prev. 11(8);777–81.

2. Novel roles of ginsenoside Rg 3 in apoptosis through downregulation of epidermal growth factor receptor. Joo EJ, et al. Chem Biol Interact. 2015.

3. Identification of molecular target of diallyl trisulfide in leukemic cells. Suda S, et al. Biosci Biotechnol Biochem. 2014.

4. Olive (Olea europea) leaf extract induces apoptosis and monocyte/macrophage differentiation in human chronic myelogenous leukemia K562 cells: insight into the underlying mechanism. Samet I, et al. Oxid Med Cell Longev. 2014.

5. Identification of licocoumarone as an apoptosis-inducing component in licorice. Watanabe M, et al. Biol Pharm Bull. 2002.

6. Aloe vera downregulates LPS-induced inflammatory cytokine production and expression of NLRP3 inflammasome in human macrophages. Budai MM, et al. Mol Immunol. 2013.

7. Green tea polyphenol epigallocatechin-0-gallate induces cell death by acid sphingomyelinase activation in chronic myeloid leukemia cells. Huang Y, et al. Oncol Rep. 2015.

8. Ethanlo extract of Hedyotis diffusa willd upregulates GO/GI phase arrest and induces apoptosis in human leukemia cells by modulating caspase cascade signaling and altering associated genes expression was assyed by cDNA microarray. Kuo YJ, et al. Environ Toxicol. 2014.

9. Increased risk of deep vein thrombosis in patients with multiple myeloma receiving thalidomide and chemotherapy. Zangari M, et al. Blood, 2001 Am Soc Hematology.

10. MiR-218 inhibits the proliferation of glioma U87 cells through the inactivation of the CDK6/cyclin D1/p21 (Cip1/Wat 1) pathway. Jun GJ, et al. Oncol Lett. 2015.

11. Current concept of photocarcinogenesis. Nishisgori C, et al. Photochem Photobiol Sci. 2015.

12. Risk of basal cell and squamous cell skin cancers after ionizing radiation therapy for the Skin Cancer Prevention Study Group. Karagas MR, et al. J Natl Cancer Inst. 1996.

13. Anticancer effect of lycopene in gastric carcinogenesis. Kim MJ, et al. J Cancer Prev. 2015.

14. European Code against Cancer 4th edition: Physical activity and cancer. Leitzmann M, et al. Cancer Epidemiol. 2015.

15. Tobacco smoke carcinogens and lung cancer. Hecht SS. J of NCI, 1999

16. The alpha-tocopherol Beta-carotene lung cancer prevention study: design, methods, participant characteristics and compliance. ATBC Cancer Prevention Study Group. Annals of Epidemiology. 1994.

17. BRCA 1 and BRCA 2 genetic testing- pitfalls and recommendations for managing variants of uncertain clinical significance. Eccles.D, et al. Ann Oncol. 2015

18. Tea consumption reduces ovarian cancer risk. Lee AH, et al. Cancer Epidemiol. 2013.

19. Circulating melatonin and the risk of breast and endometrial cancer in women. Viswanathan AN, et al. Cancer Lett, 2009.

20. Nucleoside analogs in the prevention of hepatitis B virus related hepatocellular carcinoma. Baran B, et al. World J Hepatol. 2015.

21. Inhibitory effect of genistein on PLC/PRF5 Hepatocellular Carcinoma cell line. Dastjerdi MN, et al. Int J Prev Med. 2015.

22. Cranberry phytochemicals: isolation structure elucidation and their antiproliferative and antioxidant activites. He X, et al. J Agric Food Chem 2006.

23. Conservative management and parenchyma-sparing resections of pancreatic neuroendocrine tumors. Literature review. Mauriello C, et al. Int J Surg. 2015.

24. Potential effects of pomegranate polyphenols in cancer prevention and therapy. Turrini E, et al. Oxid Med Cell Longev. 2015.

25. Lower prostate cancer risk in men with elevated plasma lycopene levels: results of a prospective analysis. Gann PH, et al. Cancer Res. 1999.

26. Sulforaphane and prostate cancer interception. Traka MH, et al. Drug Discov Today. 2014.

27. Fruit, vegetables, and cancer prevention: A review of the epidemiological evidence. Block G, et al. Nutrition and Cancer. 1992.

28. Cyclooxygenase-2 expression is upregulated in human pancreatic cancer. Tucker ON, et al. Cancer Res, Mar 1, 1999.

29. Vitamin C and cancer prevention: the epidemiologic evidence. Block G, et al. Am J Clin Nutr, Jan 1991.

30. 2'-Hydroxyflavanone: A promising molecule for kidney cancer prevention. Singhal SS, et al. Biochem Pharmacol. 2015.

31. Cancer causing prescription drugs. NEJM Sept 25, 2008.

32. Physiological aspects of male libido enhanced by standardized Trigonella foenum-graecum extract and mineral formulation. Steels E, et al. Phytother Res. 2011.

33. Panax notoginseng saponins improve erectile function through attenuation of oxidative stress, restoration of Akt activity and protection of endothelial and smooth muscle cells in diabetic rats with erectile dysfunction. Li H, et al. Urol Int. 2014.

34. Strategy to reduce free radical species in Alzheimer's disease: an update of selected antioxidants.

DiDomenico F, et al. Expert Rev Neurother. 2015 (Coenzyme Q10).

35. The role of dietary coconut for the prevention and treatment of Alzheimer's disease: potential mechanisms of action. Fernando WM, et al. Br J Nutr. 2015.

36. Caffeine: cognitive and physical performance enhancer or psychoactive drug? Cappelletti S, et al. Curr Neuropharmacol. 2015.

37. Protecting cognition from ageing and Alzheimer's disease: a computerized cognitive training combined with reminiscence therapy. Barbari F, et al. Int J Geriatr Psychiatry. 2015.

38. Fish consumption, fish oil, omega-3 fatty acids, and cardiovascular disease. Kris-Etherton, Penny M, et al. Circulation.2002;106:2747-2757 American Heart Association.

39. Stroke Risk factors: Dyken ML. Prevention of Stroke (volume) 1991, pp83–101.

40. Capsaicin and its analogues: Structure activity relationship study. Huang XF, et al. Curr Med Chem. 2013.

41. Burden of smokig among adults with COPD, chronic bronchitis, and emphysema in urban China. Goren A, et al. Int J Clin Pract. 2015.

42. Biological effects and mechanisms of action of mesenchymal stem cell therapy in chronic obstructive pulmonary disease. Jun Z, et al. J Int Med Res. 2015.

43. Cordyceps militaris alleviates severity of murine acute lung injury through miRNAs-mediated CxCR2 inhibition. Liu S, et al. Cell Physiol Biochem. 2015.

44. How effective are Antioxidant Supplements in obesity and diabetes? Abdali D, et al. Med Prin Pract. 2015 (a).

   Behavioral susceptibility to obesity: Gene environment interplay in the development of weight. Llewellyn C, et al. Physiol Behav. 2015.

45. Subclinical thyroid dysfunction and depressive symptoms among elderly: a prospective cohort study. Blum MR, et al. Neuroendocrinology. 2015.

46. Fish oil, omega03 and Crohn's disease. Cochrane database, NEJM 1996

47. Apigenin has anti-atrophic gastritis and anti-gastric cancer progression effects in Helicobacter pylori-infected Mongolian gerbils. Kuo CH, et al. J Ethnopharmacol. 2014 (chamomile).

48. A review of gastroprotective effects of ginger (Zingiber officinale Roscoe). Haniadka R, et al. Food Funct. 2013.

49. Anti-inflammatory and cytoprotective effects of selected Pakistani medicinal plants in Helicobacter pylori-infected gastric epithelial cells. Zaidi SF, et al. J Ethnopharmacol. 2012.

50. Curcumin in inflammatory disease. Shehzad A, et al. Biofactors. 2013

51. Prevention of Liver Fibrosis and cancer in Africa: The PROLIFICA project= a collaborative study of hepatitis B-related fever disease in West Africa. Howell J, et al. S Afr Med J. 2015.

52. Preventing urinary tract infections in early childhood. Williams GJ, et al. Adv Exp Med Biol. 2013.

53. Drug metabolism and pharmacokinetic diversity of Ranunculaceae medicinal compounds. Hao DC, et al. Curr Drug Metab. 2015 (black cohosh).

54. Safety and efficacy of blue cohosh (Caulophyllum Thalictroides) during pregnancy and lactation. Duguoa JJ, et al. Can J Clin Pharmacol. 2008.

55. Effect of Serenoa repens on oxidative stress, inflammatory an growth factors in obese wistar rats with benign prostatic hyperplasia. Lii Colada-Velasquez J, et al. Phytother Res. 2015.

56. Phytotherapy of benign prostatic hyperplasia. A minireview. Pagano E, et al. Phytother Res. 2014.

57. Dietary patterns after prostate cancer diagnosis in relation to disease-specific and total mortality. Yang M, et al. Cancer Prev Res (Phila). 2015

58. Antiherpes simplex virus effect of an aqueous extract of propolis. Huleihel M, et al. Isr Med Assoc J. 2002.

59. Effects of intranasal treatment with capsaicin on the recurrence of polyps after polypectomy and ethmoidectomy. Zheng C, et al. Acta Otolaryngol. 2010

60. Fish and fatty acid consumption and the risk of hearing loss in women. Curhan SG, et al. Am J Clin Nutr. 2014.

61. Age-related hearing impairment and the triad of acquired hearing loss. Yan CH, et al. Front Cell Neuro Sci. 2015.

62. Abnormal essential fatty acid composition of tissue lipids in genetically diabetic mice is partially corrected by dietary linoleic and gamma-linolenic acids. Cunname SC, et al. Br J Nutr. 1985.

63. An in-depth review on the medicinal flora Rosmarinus officinalis (Lamiaceae). Begum A, et al. Acta Sci Pol Technol Aliment. Jan-Mar 2013

64. Female androgenic alopecia, a survey of causes and therapeutic options. Duchková H, et al. Cas Lek Cash. 2015.

65. Interventions for vitiligo. Whitton ME, et al. Cochrane Database Syst Rev. 2015.

66. Traditional uses: phytochemistry and pharmacology of Ficus carica: a review. Badgujar SB, et al. Pharm Biol. 2014.

67. Biological activities of Fructus arctii fermented with the basidiomycete Grifolafrondosa. Kim JH, et al. Arch Pharm Res. 2010.

68. Antineoplastic effects of Rhodiola crenulata treatment on B16-F10 melanoma. Dudek MC. Et al. Tumour Biol. 2015.

69. Activity-guided purification identifies lupeol, a pentacyclic triterpene, as a therapeutic agent multiple pathogenic factors of acne. Kivon HH, et al. J Invest Dermatol. 2015.

70. Innovations in national ingredients and their use in skin care. Fowler JF, et al. J Drugs Dermatol. 2010.

71. Host response mechanisms in periodontal diseases. Silva N, et al. J Appl Oral Sci. 2015.

72. Association between dental caries and out-of-hospital cardiac arrests of cardiac origin in Japan. Suematou Y, et al. Cardiol. 2015.

73. Natural products for dental caries prevention. Badria FA, et al. J Med Food. 2004.

74. Pomegranate extract: a potential protector against aminoglycoside ototoxicity. Kahya V, et al. J Laryngol Otol. 2014.

75. Websites: WebMD, Medline plus Encyclopedia, CDC and Prevention, Mayo Clinic Disease Prevention, Med Journal articles published (PubMed), Dental Health Foundation, American Medical Association.

Index

Appendix

Antibiotic Foods

Onions and garlic: contain organosulfur compounds

Honey: contains methylglyoxal activity against bacteria associated with sore throat

Cabbage, broccoli, kale, cauliflower (cruciferous vegetables)

Probiotics (fermented good bacteria)

Grapefruit seeds (extract) bactericidal

Cranberry (prevents bacterial adherence to mucosal bladder lining)

Pomegranate (bactericidal, kills E.coli, Bacillus cereus, Staph aureus)

Inflammation Control Diet

Omega 3 fish oils (or capsules 1,000mg): avoid or restrict

Flaxseed oil (capsules or seeds) safflower, sunflower, Crisco, butter, beans, legumes, wild salmon margarine, vegetable oils

Antioxidants fried foods:

fruits, vegetables, berries fast foods

salmon, sardines, walnuts dairy products

Whole foods animal protein

Fiber (whole wheat, cracked grain) red meat, yeast

Soy (iron, calcium, protein, vit. B12) white sugar

Green tea excess alcohol,

Olive oil (extra virgin) refined carbohydrates

Canola oil (cooking) tobacco

Garlic and onions processed wheat

Calcium (broccoli, collards, juices, kale) caffeine, peanuts, gluten

Iron (chickpeas, pinto beans, spinach) polyunsaturated vegetable oils

Vitamin B12 (corn, legumes, beans, peanuts, margarine, soy, rice, pasta, whole wheat, bread)

Botanicals

Ginger, Turmeric, Cayenne

Evening primrose oil,

Boswellia, Cat's claw,

Devil's claw, cayenne,

Chamomile, tylophora

Antioxidants

Vitamin C **blueberry**

Vitamin A (beta carotene) beans

Vitamin E **cranberry, blackberry**

Vitamin D artichoke, raisins

Bilberry **strawberry**

Lutein **apple (**granny smith and red delicious)

Zeaxanthin pecan

Zinc potato

Selenium **cherry, raspberry**

Cayenne **plum, prunes**

Turmeric dates

Ginger avocado

Coenzyme Q10 pear

Bioflavonoids (tomatoes, spinach, grapefruit, guava, broccoli, grapes, red wine)

Isoflavones (soy, legumes, beans, berries)

Carotenoids (red, green, and orange vegetables: carrots, sweet potatoes, dark leafy greens, tomatoes, squash—lycopene, lutein…skin, bones, immune system)

Celery macadamia and all nuts

Green tea asparagus

Quercetin grapefruit, apricot

Suma banana

Kutaki pepper

Cat's claw peach

Cantaloupe, melon, grapes, kiwi, mango, nectarine, orange, tangerine, watermelon

Cabbage corn

Carrot cucumber

Cauliflower onion, peas, lettuce, eggplant

Anti-Cancer Foods

Need large amounts in order for the phytochemicals to be effective in established cancer. Most effective when consumed four to six servings a day on a regular basis and for purposes of prevention.

1. Almonds *(Prunus dulcis)*: protease inhibitors, phytate, genistein, lignans,

2. *Amaranth (Amaranthus* retroflexus): greens (folic acid, carotenes, calcium) Grains/seeds (protein, lignans, protease inhibitors)

3. Apples (*Malus communis*): chlorogenic and caffeic acids, apple cider vinegar

4. Apricots (*Armeniaca vulgaris*): pits have laetrile (amyygdalin, vit. B17, cyanide)

5. Barley (*Hordeum vulgare*) protease inhibitors, carotenes

6. Beans (*Phaseolus vulgaris*) dried (soak overnight and discard water before cooking

7. Beets (*Beta rubra*): strengthen immunity and kills cancer cells

8. Bok choy *(Brassica chinensis)* cytotoxic

9. Broccoli (*Brassica oleracea*): protease inhibitors blocks cancer initiation and inhibits side effects of radiation; lutein, indoles, sulforaphane, glucosinolates, dithiolthiones…

10. Brussels Sprouts (*Brassica oleracea*): same as cabbage, collards, cauliflower, kale

11. Burdock root (*Arctium lappa*).. vs cancers initiated by chemicals and radiation

12. Cabbage: antioxidant; best when cooked as sauerkraut

13.   Carrots (*Daucus carota*) beta carotenes, carotenoids, chlorogenic acids; has asparagin, resists radiation damage

14.   Cauliflower (*Brassica oleracea*)..indoles, sulforaphane

15.   Celery (*Apium graveolens*)… antioxidants, folic acid, mineral salts, build
   RBC's, adrenals

16.   Cereal grasses: wheat , rye, barley, rice, oatstraw

17.   Chickpeas *(Cicer arietinum*): protease inhibitors, Garbanzo beans

18.   Corn (*Zea mays*): rich in protease inhibitors and influences thyroid hormone output…

19.   Figs (*Ficus carica*): anticancer phytochemical benza-ldehyde (injections of distillate and poultices used in Japanese hospitals)

20.   Flaxseed (*Linum usitatissimum*): anticancer lignans, gallic acid, ferulic acid

21.   Garlic (*Allium sativum*): inhibits growth of breast cancer cells…

22.   Ginger (*Zingiber off*) antioxidants and carotenes; anti-inflammation

23.   Grapes (*Vinis vinifera*) selenium, trace minerals, ellagic acid, tannins, caffeic acid…

24.   Grapefruit (*Citrus paradis*) pectin, linalool, naringens

25. Green tea (*Camilla sinensis*): epigallocatechins

26. Horseradiash (*Amoracia rusticana*): anticancer acids (carbonic, silicic, phosphatic, sulfuric, hydrochloric acid)

27. Lemon (*Citrus major*): citronella, limonene

28. Lentils (*Lens culinaris*): protease inhibitors, genistein, lignans...repair of damaged DNA

29. Moringa (*M. oleifera*) polyphenols, amino acids, vitamins, minerals, zeatin, moringa YSP (immunomodulatory), niazimicin and kaempferol (cytotoxic)

30. Millet (*Panicum milliaceum*): Africa staple...source of laetrile, protease inhibitors, lignans, carotenes

31. Canola oil (*Brassica napus*): from seeds of cabbage plant

32. Olive oil (*Olea europaea*): resists rancidity, antioxidant

33. Sesame oil (*Sesamum indicum*): tahini, antioxidants, lignana, phenols

34. Onion (*Allium cepa*): can reverse cellular changes that cause cancer

35. Orange peels: antioxidants, flavonoids, triterpenoids, limonene

36. Parsley (*Petroselinum crispum*): carotenes, vit. C, folic acid, chlorophyll

37. Pineapple (*Ananas comosus*): bromelain digestive enzyme, reduces prostaglandin production (anti-inflammatory)

38. Pomegranate (*Punica granatum*): ellagitannin, granatin B, vit. C, protease inhibitors

39. Potatoes (*Solanum tuberosum*): protease inhibitors, polyphenols

40. Purslane (*Portulaca oleracea*) antioxidants, carotenes, folic acid, omega-3 , glutathione

41. Radishes (*Raphanus sativus*): daikon, exceptional anticancer, used in Chinese hospitals

42. Rhubarb (*Rheum rhaponticum*): stalks, cooked

43. Seasoning herbs: mints, turmeric, .anti-inflammation

44. Seaweed, soy beans (*Soya hispida*)

45. Soursop (*Annona muricata*): graviola, annonacin, acetogenins, betastilbesterol, stearic, myristic acids

46. Stinging nettle: richest source of carotenes and chlorophyll; good for chemo

47. Turnips (*Brassica rapa*): roots and greens

48. Watercress (*Nasturtium off*)

49. Wild mushrooms: puffballs (Calvatia), reishii (*Ganoderma lucidum*), oyster m. (*Pleurotus ostreatus*), shiitake (*Lentinus edodes*), straw m. (*Volvariella volva-*

cea). Maitake (*Grifolia frondosa*), Zhu ling (*Polyporus umbellatus*), chaga (*Inonotus obliquus*)

50. Yogurt: a quart a week…

Best Foods for Disease Prevention

Fruit: antioxidants, vitamins, and fiber

Blueberry, raspberry
Guava, pomegranate
Apples, avocado
Cranberry, citrus
Coconut

Vegetables: Kale, broccoli, spinach, asparagus, artichokes, radish

Mushrooms: Shiitake, maitake
Garlic, onions, leeks
Sweet potatoes, eggplant

Herbs: Ginger, turmeric

Moringa, green tea

Protein: Salmon, sardines, tuna

Flaxseed, lean red meat
Beans: soybeans
Eggs, sulfur
Mixed nuts: walnuts, almonds

Roquefort cheese
Oats, cereals
Yogurt

Carbohydrates: Chocolate fruit

Cholesterol Management

Decrease saturated fats and high cholesterol food intake.

Vegetables, parsley, artichokes, no trans-fats or partially hydrated oils

Whole grains, cereals

Oatmeal, tofu, soy

Garlic (one clove, uncooked, daily) or capsules

Quit smoking.

Flaxseed oil

Red wine

Walnuts, olive oil

Fish (sardines, salmon, cod, tuna)

Fiber (beans, barley, lentils, citrus, peas, carrots)

Supplements:

Shiitake mushrooms

Vitamin B3 (Niacin) bid

Green tea (*prevents cholesterol from oxidizing*)

Guggul, 1,000mg t.i.d. or Kutaki (*picorrhiza*), 100 mg daily

Omega-3 capsules, 1,000mg daily

Red yeast rice, 1,200mg twice a day

Cholesterol essentials daily (soy, niacin, vitamin C, coenzyme Q10)

Exercise:

Maintain ideal body weight (*see exercise guidelines*).

Exercise Guidelines

Burn fat:

Timing: Exercise in the morning

Warm up: 5 to 10 minutes stretching (increase temperature, circulation, heart rate)

Intensity: low intensity to sustained period of time

Duration: 20 to 30 minutes

Action: uses carbohydrates for energy in first few minutes then uses stored fat calories

Training zone:

Fat burned: 130, 125, 118, 110, 100 calories

Age: 40, 50, 60, 70, 80

Aerobic exercise: requires large amounts of oxygen for prolonged period of time

Strengthen the cardiovascular system

Higher training zone/ heart rate range

Aerobic: 155, 145, 140, 130, 125, 115

Age: 30, 40, 50, 60, 70, 80

Start slowly, X weeks, then

Exercise 20 to 30 minutes with your heart rate in your training zone

Breathe regularly and deeply as you exercise: *never* hold your breath

Cool down/ finish with 5 to 10 minutes of stretching (flexibility)

Burn calories:

Timing: exercise in the evening (eliminate what you took in that day)

Intensity: moderate

Duration: 20 to 30 minutes

Action: uses up calories taken in that day, then stored fat

Water Regimen

8-ounce glass or stainless steel thermos or 10-ounce water bottle (Do not freeze or reuse plastic water bottles; be aware of BPA and/or BPS toxins in the plastic.)

1. Drink 8 ounces water upon awakening, first thing.

2. Water at breakfast

3. Water before starting activity or before starting work

4. Water at mid-morning break

5. Water at lunch

6. Water at tea time or at the four o'clock break

7. Water before dinner

8. Water after dinner

Drink water every time get into a car and before exiting the car.

Keep thermos of water in the car; do not go home unless it is empty.

Refill immediately.

Formula to achieve hydration by body weight:

.5 ounces × body weight (pounds) = daily requirement of water

.5 × 140 lbs = 70 ounces of water needed

1 glass, 8 ounces, therefore, you need 8 1/2 to 9 glasses per day

.5 ounces × 180 lbs = 90 ounces, 11 glasses water per day

Foods for Specific Organ Systems

Heart

Barley, blueberries

Pinto beans, broccoli

Grapes, salmon/sardines

Macadamia nuts, walnuts

Mineral water *(contains magnesium and calcium to help with blood pressure control)*

Bones

Lean top sirloin, 4 oz. *(has zinc 8mg = bone protecting; Alaska King crab 10mg zinc)*

Broccoli and spinach *(Vitamin K -> transports calcium/ metabolize it into bone)*

Digestion

Blueberries *(anthocyanins, decreased risk of colon cancer)*

Also cherries, strawberries, concord grapes

Popcorn (air popped) *is an insoluble fiber, assists peristalsis)*

Bananas (*protease inhibitors to fight off H.pylori* bacteria)

Avoid refined or processed foods, which lead to blood pressure spikes

Vision

Leafy greens (lutein, zeaxanthin = carotenoids) help absorb UV, protect retina, reduce cataract formation; betacarotente = fat soluble therefore must cook the greens first (steam or bake) then add olive oil to maximize absorption; low-fat milk with riboflavin (B2) prevent cataracts (helps manufacture glutathione which fights free radicals) fortified milk with vitamin D3 reduces macular degeneration.

Breast Cancer Protection

Cauliflower (cruciferous) with sulforaphene (*stops cancer cells from reproducing*) has I3C (lowers estrogen levels)

Vegetables: roast or steam (do not boil, as they lose 75 percent of cancer-fighting compounds into the water)

Sweet potatoes: beta-carotene (helps metabolize estrogen)

Tomato sauce: Lycopene: antioxidant—free radicals suppression; is fat soluble, therefore add olive oil to help absorption

Nuts and seeds reduce inflammation and promote tissue repair.

Discontinue grapefruit after menopause as it interacts with estrogen and increases its potency

Lungs

Pears and apples: quercetin (flavonoid), decrease risk of asthma

Edamame: (phytoestrogens), tofu, lentils

Brown rice: selenium vs. free radicals; whole wheat bread, chicken, eggs

Joints (Arthritis)

Olive oil (omega 3), oranges (vitamin C)

Memory

Apples (acetylcholine, antioxidants)

Chicken breast (niacin) 14mg/d; roast, skinless with herbs

Yellowfin tuna, salmon

Coffee (reduces Alzheimer's by 65 percent) decreases saturated and trans fats

Skin

Light tuna (selenium) protects against sun damage, 55mg turkey

Fortified instant cereal dark chocolate (high flavonoids)

Black tea with citrus (flavonoids and polyphenols), carrot juice (betacarotene)

Sources of Essential Vitamins and Minerals

Omega 3: cold-water fish oils salmon (fresh Pacific), sardines, mackerel, herring, swordfish, shrimp, albacore tuna, soy, yogurt, butter, eggs, flaxseed, walnuts, olive oil, canola oil, with DHA, EPA, ALA, GLA, Borage oil *(most disease is due to a diet high in fat and low in fiber; with excess toxins)*

Lutein and Zeaxanthin: melons, blueberries, pears, grapes, peach, plum, strawberries

Vitamin A: carrots, cantaloupes, sweet potatoes, spinach, kale, tomatoes, papaya milk, cereals, broccoli, mango, apricots (beta-carotene, not retinol), 10,000 to 15,000 IU

Vitamin B6: pyroxidine, wheat bran, yeast, molds, soy, lecithin, bananas, carrots, lentils, tuna, salmon, sunflower seeds, 25 to 50mg

Vitamin C: citrus, carambolas, acerolas, mango, guava, lemon (master cleanser) lime, kiwi, 500 to1000mg

Vitamin D: calciferol 3, made in the skin due to UV-B/ Ca metabolism with Mg; bones

Cod liver oil, fortified milk and orange juice, coldwater fish, sunlight 800 to 1200 IU

Vitamin E: mayonnaise, salad dressings, cereals, grains, cold-pressed olive oil, vegetable oils, sunflower seeds, avocados, almonds, hazelnuts, walnuts, wheat germ, 400 to 800 IU

Folate: cereal, yeast, bread, orange juice, dried beans, lentils, 400 to 600mcg

Copper: oysters, shellfish, grains, beans, nuts, potatoes, organ meats, dark leafy greens, dried fruits, cocoa, black pepper, 900mcg

Selenium: Brazil nuts, organ meats, fish, shellfish, chicken, wheat germ, brewer's yeast, 80 to 200mcg

Zinc: oysters, turkey (dark meat), eggs, pumpkins seeds, crabmeat, yogurt, milk, beans, nuts, 15mg

Food Sources of Basic Nutrients (US Diet)

Fat: Beef, margarine, salad dressing, mayonnaise, cheese, milk

Protein: Beef, poultry, milk, yeast bread, cheese

Carbohydrates: yeast bread, sodas, cookies/cakes, sugar/syrup/jam, potatoes

Fiber: yeast, wheat bread, cereal, beer (0.7g fiber per 12 ounces), carrots

Vitamins:

A: carrots, cereal, milk, margarine, organ meats

C: orange juice, grapefruit juice,

E: mayonnaise, salad dressing, cereals

Calcium: milk, cheese, yeast bread, ice cream, yogurt, cakes/cookies

Folate: cereal, yeast bread, orange juice, dried beans, and lentils

Energy sources: yeast bread, meat, sugars, alcohol, cereals

Cholesterol: eggs, beef, poultry, milk, cheese

Monounsaturated fat: omega-3 fatty acids, olive oil, canola oil

Polyunsaturated fat: salad dressing, mayonnaise, margarine

Saturated fat: cheese, beef, milk, hot dogs

Immune System Enhancing Foods

Cruciferous Vegetables: arugula, horseradish

Bokchoy, kale

Broccoli, kohlrabi

Broccolini, mustard greens

Brussels sprouts, radishes

Cabbage, red cabbage

Cauliflower, turnip, greens

Collards, watercress

Anti-angiogenic foods (stop or prevent formation of new blood vessels that leak)

Onions and garlic (allium vegetables), omega 3 fats (olive oil, fish)

Berries (all), peppers

Black rice, pomegranate

Cinnamon, quince

Citrus, resveratrol (from grapes and red wine)

Cruciferous vegetables, soybeans

Flaxseeds, spinach

Ginger, tomatoes (lycopene)

Green tea, turmeric

Mushrooms (medicinal = maitake, shiitake, reischi); seeds (chia, sesame, sunflower)

Natural Estrogen Rreplacement

For menopause (estradiol, estrone, estriol)

Black cohosh: hot flashes; "similar" to estrogen, use for six months or with progesterone,

Capsules, 20 to 80mg twice daily

Dong quai root: menstrual cycle regulation and pain control, no estrogen activity = a tonic; 200 mg three times a day or 3.5 to 4.0 grams/day. As it is a "heating" herb, it may cause hot flashes, insomnia, etc.

Vitex: for early menopause and dysmenorrhea, mastalgia

Wild yams (cream without alcohol, natural dascheen, roots, tania,ñamé, yucca)

Papaya, phytoestrogens (daily)

Pomegranates

Red clover: Promensil 40 mg; *not* for menopause as it simulates estradiol effect on cell proliferation in breast cancer cells but is good for skin and respiratory ailments

Omega 3 fish oil (DHA and EPA): effects on cholesterol, endocrine function

Evening primrose oil (GLA)

Vit E: hot flashes, reduced breast cancer chances, 800 IU daily

Shepherd's purse: staunches flow of blood (hemostasis), menorrhagia, metiorrhagia

Phytoestrogens: isoflavones phytosterols lignans

Soy beans 100mg/day (plant-based) seeds

Legumes, papaya fruit

Chickpeas, vegetables

Pinto beans, whole grains

Lima beans

Alfalfa

Acupuncture: alleviation of hot flashes and most menopausal symptoms

Answers to Self-Assessment Questionnaire

(See chapter 1.)

1. Longevity owes some credence to genetics but mostly to environment and the lifestyle choices of the individual. Regular exercise, a healthy balanced diet, social connections, mental stimulation, stress control, and avoidance of exposure to toxins and risky behavior, have all proven to extend the length and quality of human life.

2. A diet rich in antioxidants (berries, fruit, vegetables, monounsaturated fats, fiber), regular physical activity for blood circulation, and avoidance of exposure to toxins all contribute to maintaining the health of sense organs.

3. Most pharmaceutical drugs are synthetic and consist of chemicals with one or two mechanisms of action designed to suppress of stimulate a specific target. They are usually devoid of balance and so result in unwanted side effects. Whole food and plants with medicinal properties, though slower in onset, are more balanced and directed toward prevention of disease.

4. Maintaining good health through regular good life-style choices is the best way to avoid debilitating bankrupting disease.

5. Traveling in a foreign country provides your body with challenges to which it is not accustomed. A healthy functional immune system is one way to handle exposure to invasive organisms. Avoidance of endemic areas, contaminated water, and precautions against mosquitoes are basic. Knowledge of the environment and precautionary measures are recommended.

6. Overexposure to UV radiation from the sun can and will cause skin cancers in susceptible individuals. One can get adequate vitamin D from fifteen minutes sun exposure per day—not enough to give skin cancer. Total avoidance of sunlight may lead to vitamin D deficiency.

7. A fully balanced diet of protein, fats, and carbohydrates contributes to the prevention of disease. The intake of plant-based protein, some lean meat, omega-3 cold water fish, flaxseed, beans, legumes, fresh green vegetables, fruit, whole grains, fiber, olive oil, berries, nuts and seeds, and the avoidance of processed, refined, chemically treated foods will greatly contribute to good health.

8. Genetics accounts for about 10 to 20 percent of disease susceptibility in some cases. Lifestyle choices in the food we eat, physical activity levels, amount of stress and how it is handled, and exposure to toxins are all trigger mechanisms that can set off and maintain progression of a particular disease.

9. Dementia and its various forms like Alzheimers can be prevented or delayed by continued mental stimulation, exercise to increase blood flow and oxygen to the brain cells, eating a balanced diet high in protective antioxidants, omega-3 foods, anti-inflammation foods, and specifics like coconut oil, which have been shown to supply the brain with energy.

10. Cholesterol control is a balance between high density (good) and low density (bad) forms. Good fats like avocado and extra virgin olive oil can raise HDL levels while trans fats and polyunsaturated fats raise the LDL. Natural foods like bran, oats, green tea, ginger, fiber, beans, lentils, soy, flaxseed, and barley are known to help lower LDL cholesterol. Be aware of the long-term use of statins and their side effects.

11. Weight control and avoidance of obesity depends on several basic strategies. Decrease portion size of each food group to the amount that fits in the palm of your hand; four to five small meals a day are better than three big ones; eat low-glycemic foods; avoid

fast foods, packaged foods, trans fats, chips, cookies, commercially baked goods, sodas, and sugar-laced energy drinks. Exercise to burn fat and keep the weight off.

12. Dietary supplements can be good when traveling or living in a region where availability of whole fresh organic food is lacking. Be sure to read the label and use a reputable brand. Whole food is always better than supplements.

13. Read the labels or skin care products very carefully and avoid too many artificial chemicals. Essential fatty acids have anti-inflammatory properties, support natural defenses of skin, support the natural aging process, and promote healthy skin without covering it up. Note that vitamin D is essential. Get some sun.

14. Differences in health of a given group of people depend on a combination of factors. A strong functional immune system built on the principles of good basic lifestyle strategies appears to be a very important factor in health vs. disease.

15. GMOs (genetically modified organisms) are used to produce food crops (eg. corn, soy) that are resistant to the pesticides that are applied in order to increase and ensure high yields. A new genetic sequence is injected into a one-celled animal. All adult cells will

have the new sequence, usually one of resistance and blockage. The effects on humans after consumption are as yet unknown. General consensus is that it is "unnatural" and should not be used. The fact is that harmful pesticides are still used in their production.

Be aware that recombinant bovine growth hormone is proven to be bad for health but gives more meat, higher profits, results in poorer health and ultimately higher costs of health care.

16. Cancer prevention can be achieved through a diet high in antioxidant foods, intake of specific botanicals (eg. green tea), exercise, avoidance of bad food and exposure to toxins, and reduction and control of stress.

About the Author

Alfred L. Anduze is a retired physician, past assistant commissioner of Health, president of the Ophthalmic Society of West Indies, Ophthalmology Consultants of USVI, Atlanta Ophthalmology Consultants; assistant professor of Ophthalmology University of Florida, Jacksonville, Editorial Board of Annals of Ophthalmology; and lecturer in thirty-two countries. Having published three medical textbooks, seventeen ophthalmic journal articles, seven articles on health and nature, and five Caribbean books, and holding an Andrew Weil Fellowship in Integrative Medicine and a master's certificate in herbal medicine, he retired in 2012 and moved up to farming. With a chief interest in biology, botany, and biochemistry as they apply to aging, natural health, and preventive medicine, he currently works with his wife at Saluan Farm Health and Wellness Center in Maricao, Puerto Rico.

> I spent 40 years learning and practicing western medicine's brand of diagnosis after the fact, then dispensing toxic drugs and performing body altering surgery. I expect to spend the next 40 years learning, practicing and teaching preventive medicine using basic natural tenets, exercise, nutritional, energy and

mind-body principles, stress and inflammation control and a better understanding and implementation of social interactions. (Alfred L. Anduze, MD)

CPSIA information can be obtained
at www.ICGtesting.com
Printed in the USA
FSOW03n2047061016
25778FS